the right carb

First published in the United Kingdom in 2021 by
Pavilion
43 Great Ormond Street
London
WC1N 3HZ

Copyright © Pavilion Books Company Ltd 2021
Text copyright © Nicola Graimes 2021

ISBN 978-1-91166-320-1

A CIP catalogue record for this book is available from the British Library.
10 9 8 7 6 5 4 3 2 1

Reproduction by Rival Colour Ltd., UK
Printed and bound by Toppan Leefung Ltd, China
www.pavilionbooks.com

Publisher: Helen Lewis
Photographer: Haarala Hamilton
Food stylist: Valerie Berry
Props stylist: Rachel Vere
Project editor: Sophie Allen
Design manager: Laura Russell
Design layout: Hannah Naughton
Illustrations: Nick Paul Jordan
Recipe analysis: Alina Tierney
Production manager: Phil Brown

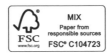

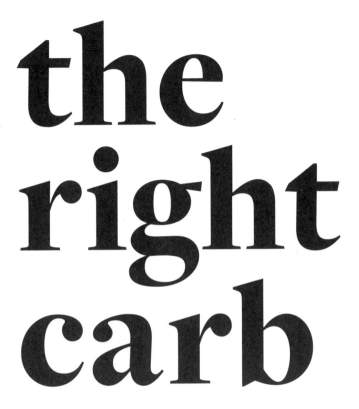

the right carb

How to enjoy carbs with over 50 simple, nutritious recipes for good health

Nicola Graimes

PAVILION

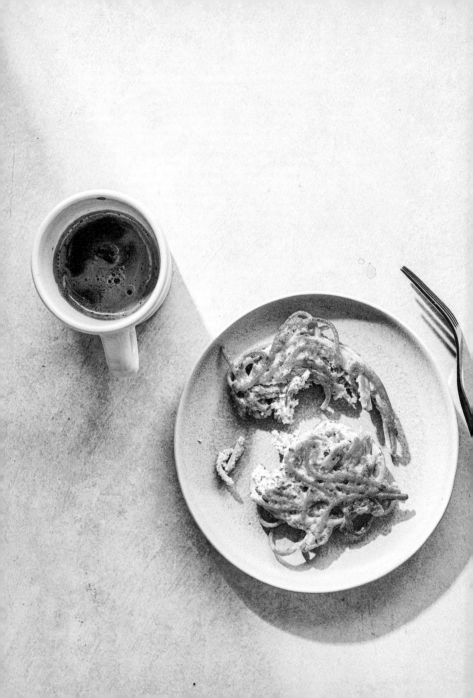

Speaking up for Carbs

Carbohydrate has almost become a dirty word, so you may well ask why I have written a book celebrating this much-maligned food group. In recent years, the role of carbs in our diet and their effect on our health has become a bit of a hot potato, excuse the pun. Everyone seems to have a strong opinion on carbs and much of it is steeped in confusion.

The more I learn about carbs – our body's main and preferred source of energy – the more I want to stand up for them. Yet, I'm more than well aware that not all carbohydrates are created equal: while some come with a whole host of health attributes – let's call them the 'right' carbs – there are others that offer very little; they have even been labelled nutritionally void. In the right camp are wholegrains, pulses (peas, beans and lentils), fruit, vegetables and nuts and seeds. This book is a celebration of these fine foods, not only of their many health benefits but also of their incredible diversity and the joy they bring to our cooking and eating.

The Right Carb cookbook concentrates on the positive effects of eating the right carbs, from reducing the risk of heart disease, type 2 diabetes and bowel cancer to supporting the health of the gut, boosting mood and aiding sleep. It shows how to shop for the right carbs as well as the best ways to prepare and cook them for maximum enjoyment and nutrition. These recipes show that by combining the right carbs with other food groups, primarily good-quality plant proteins, small amounts of animal protein and good fats, you can create delicious, nutritious meals.

Don't get me wrong, I'm not advocating bingeing on doughnuts, eating humungous bowls of white rice or splurging on crisps, but this book is in response to everyone who has dismissed carbs as the 'bad guys'. It shows that eating the right carbs in the right amounts can contribute to the long-term health of body and mind – and the pleasure of great, tasty food. It's time to change how we look at carbohydrates and revive our enjoyment of this valuable food group.

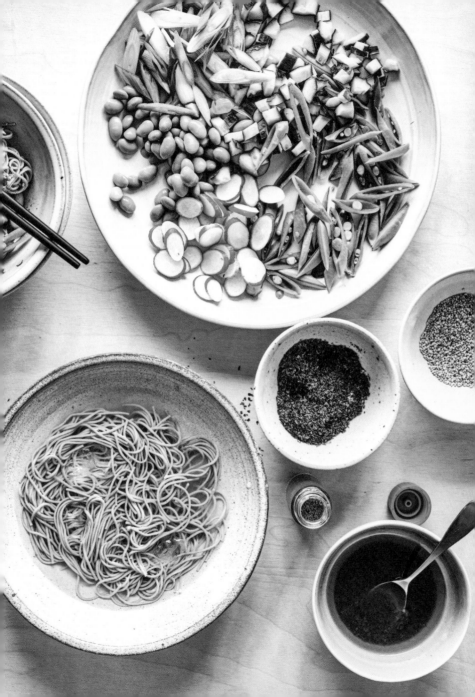

About the Recipes

The Right Carb cookbook is all about eating well for long-term good health, rather than a punishing regime or diet. There are over 50 simple everyday recipes using whole, unrefined carbohydrates – think pulses, wholegrains, nuts, seeds, fruit and vegetables – combined with predominantly plant-based protein and good fats. I've included a handful of recipes featuring meat in small, sustainable amounts. You'll also find a few fish and seafood recipes to add balance.

There are recipes for all types of meal and occasion. Breakfast is often high in refined carbs – think cereal, toast, fruit juice – but it doesn't have to be if you include a mix of wholegrains, beans and vegetables, and balance the carb element with a protein food like eggs or yogurt. Likewise, a side dish of mashed potatoes, white rice or pasta can be transformed into a right carb one by swapping these with fibre-rich whole versions. You'll also find ideas for light meals, many of which would make a healthy packed lunch, alongside more substantial recipes for complete meals.

The desserts all use fruit rather than added sugar, honey or maple syrup. For me, this is the best way to add sweetness as you also reap its nutritional benefits. Even bananas – one of the higher-carb/high GI fruits – are excellent for adding sweetness as well as texture and flavour to cakes, bakes and ice creams. Dried fruit is higher in sugar than fresh, but it comes with more fibre and a higher concentration of vitamins and minerals. Small amounts of dried fruit make a delicious treat and when eaten with protein and/or healthy fats, such as Greek-style yogurt, nuts and seeds, they have less of an impact on blood sugar levels than when eaten on their own, and are more filling.

The Bigger Picture

The focus of this book is on the right carbs, but it's also vital to look at the bigger picture, which means our diets as a whole, rather than one food group in isolation. Hand-in-hand with the right carbs come the other macronutrients, proteins and fats, which work in tandem to support our health. Protein is made up of amino acids, some of which our bodies are able to produce and nine of which we have to get from food. With the exception of soya beans, quinoa, buckwheat and amaranth, which are complete proteins (they contain all nine essential amino acids), most plant-based foods are lacking in some amino acids. However, nature is clever: eating a varied diet containing both protein and carbs on a daily basis, not necessarily at every meal, ensures that you get all the amino acids you need.

Factor in too that most foods are made up of a combination of macro-nutrients. Pulses, for instance, may be known for their impressive right carb and fibre content, but they are also relatively high in protein and contain small amounts of fat, making them an especially healthy addition to your diet.

Right Carbs – What are they?

There are two main types of carbohydrate – simple and complex. Simple carbohydrates are basically sugars, which are broken down quickly leading to unstable blood sugar levels and are best avoided. Complex carbohydrates are made up of plant-based starches and fibre. These provide a steady release of energy depending on how close the food is to its natural, unprocessed state. Generally, the less processed the food, the slower the release of energy, the higher its nutritional value and the better it is for you.

Thumbs-up to the right carbs:

- **Wholegrains:** barley, spelt, buckwheat, quinoa, brown rice, black rice, Camargue red rice, brown jasmine rice, oats, rye, amaranth, wholewheat.

- **Beans and pulses:** chickpeas, red kidney beans, cannellini beans, haricot beans, butter (lima) beans, black-eyed beans (peas), flageolet beans, aduki (adzuki) beans, black beans, green, brown, red and Puy lentils.

- **Peas:** marrowfat, split and whole yellow peas, split green peas, carlin.

- **Vegetables (starchy):** potatoes (in their skin), sweet potatoes (in their skin), squash, pumpkin, carrots, parsnips, celeriac (celery root), swede (rutabaga), parsnips, Jerusalem artichokes (sunchokes).

- **Vegetables (non-starchy):** red (bell) peppers, broccoli, asparagus, mushrooms, courgettes (zucchini), spinach, cauliflower, green beans, salad leaves, kale and cavolo nero, cucumber, celery, tomatoes, radishes, onions, aubergine (eggplant), cabbage, globe artichokes, Swiss chard.

- **Fruit:** strawberries, raspberries, blueberries, blackberries, grapefruit, apricots, peaches, nectarines, lemon, kiwis, oranges, melon, apples, bananas, pears.

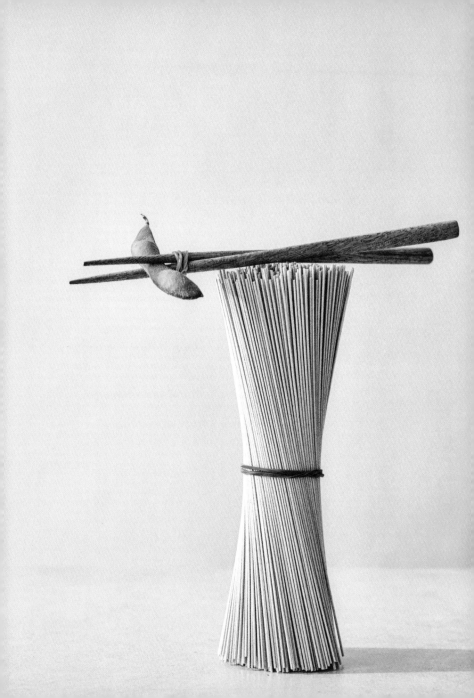

The Glycaemic Index (GI)

For some dieticians, labelling foods simple or complex is too simplistic, hence the use of the Glycaemic Index (GI). This ranks foods from 0 to 100 to measure how quickly a food turns to glucose in the blood (pure glucose is rated 100). White bread, sugar and fruit juice have a high GI, while brown rice, beans and lentils have a low GI.

There are, however, factors that can influence a food's GI. Serving a carb with protein or fat – a baked potato with beans and cheese, for instance – will reduce the overall GI. That's because both protein and fat slow down the digestion and absorption of carbohydrates and produce a smaller rise in blood sugar levels than if the potato was eaten on its own. Similarly, foods that are high in fibre do not cause a large spike in blood sugar levels.

What are the Wrong Carbs?

It may be too simplistic to split carbohydrates into 'right' and 'wrong' – and I use the term 'wrong' lightly – but there's no denying that highly processed foods, including sugar, cakes, biscuits, white rice, white flour and fruit drinks, are lacking in nutritional value – however lovely they may taste. These are 'empty' carbs that may lead to a list of health problems, including an increased risk of type 2 diabetes, heart disease, cancer and obesity.

When it comes to good health, it is the amount and quality of the carbs you eat that matters. Switching to a diet based on wholegrains, pulses, vegetables and fruit will provide long-term, sustained amounts of energy and ensure you get the fibre, vitamins and minerals you need.

Watch out for hidden refined carbs, too. Sugar, in particular, can crop up in the most unlikely places, such as salad dressings, sushi, bread, canned vegetables, processed meats, soup, plain yogurt, dairy-free milk, crackers and oatcakes. So-called 'healthy' cereal bars often contain an inordinate amount of sugar, and the same goes for many processed low-fat foods where the fat is often replaced by sugar to add bulk and flavour.

Sugar by Another Name...

Sugar comes under a number of guises and it pays to check food labels – you may be surprised to find that some packaged foods contain not just one, but a number of the following sugars:

- Sucrose
- Fructose
- Glucose
- Dextrose
- High-fructose glucose syrup

- Levulose
- Invert sugar
- Corn syrup/sugar
- Isoglucose
- Maltose

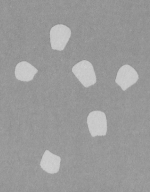

How Much is 'Right'?

While there are general guidelines, an individual's optimal carb intake is influenced by a number of factors, including sex, age, body composition, genetics, activity levels and metabolic health.

That said, a recent US study on Dietary Carbohydrate Intake and Mortality published in *The Lancet* in 2018 reached the conclusion that a diet featuring a moderate amount of carbs (around 50–55 per cent of calories), rather than extremely low (below 40 per cent) or high (over 70 per cent) is best for our long-term health and well-being, with either extreme said to negatively affect life expectancy.

Guidelines on recommended carb intake range between 225–325g/8–11½ oz for someone eating 2,000 calories per day (so 275g/9¾ oz would be considered moderate). Translating this to a plate of food: roughly 50 per cent of calories should come from carbs (half from starchy veg/grains/pulses and the other half from non-starchy vegetables); 25 per cent from good-quality protein (mainly plant-based); and 25 per cent from healthy fats. This breakdown is slightly less than the Eat Well UK government guidelines, which recommends that a third of our diet should come from starchy foods and another third from fruit and vegetables with the remaining third split between protein and fat.

What's a portion/serving?

- 1 slice wholewheat, rye or buckwheat bread
- 1 small–medium fruit or handful of berries
- 1 medium baked potato
- 1 corn on the cob
- 4–5 tbsp whole uncooked oats or other grains
- ½ x 400g (14 oz) can beans, lentils or pulses

The Wonders of Fibre

The real star of right-carb eating is fibre. There is strong evidence that a high-fibre diet can reduce the risk of heart disease, bowel cancer, strokes and type 2 diabetes. Furthermore, it keeps the gut healthy by encouraging the passage of food through the digestive system, keeping us regular and preventing constipation, as well as supporting and feeding 'friendly' gut bacteria.

The main issue with fibre is that most of us don't eat enough. According to the UK Scientific Advisory Committee on Nutrition 2015 *Carbohydrates and Health Report*, adults should be getting about 30g/1 oz of fibre a day, which is considerably more than the 19g/¾ oz per day many of us are actually eating.

I've suggested ways to increase your fibre intake below, but remember to do this gradually, making sure you drink enough fluids (around 6–8 glasses a day for adults), otherwise it may put a strain on your digestive system, which can lead to bloating and wind and aggravate conditions like irritable bowel syndrome (IBS).

How Much Fibre?
(How to reach 30g/1 oz per day)

1 (unpeeled) pear: 5.5g

½ avocado: 5g

1 banana: 2.5g

100g wholewheat pasta: 4.5g

100g carrots: 2.8g

100g broccoli: 3g

100g lentils: 8g

100g kidney beans: 6.5g

100g chickpeas: 7.6g

100g black beans: 8.7 g

100g quinoa: 2.8 g

100g oats: 10.6 g

100g popcorn: 14.5 g

100g (unblanched) whole almonds: 12.5g

100g (unpeeled) sweet potatoes: 2.5g

100g dark chocolate (70% cocoa solids): 11g

Easy ways to increase fibre in your diet:

- Snack on nuts and seeds.

- Stick to wholegrains, such as brown rice, oats, barley, rye, buckwheat and spelt.

- Try unsweetened soya (soy), oat or nut milk with wholegrain, no-added-sugar breakfast cereals.

- Add beans and lentils to salads, stews and soups.

- Top porridge with fresh or dried fruit and nuts/seeds.

- Serve potatoes and sweet potatoes in their skins with beans and cheese.

- Top wholewheat bread or toast with nut butter and sliced apple (unpeeled).

- Pop your own popcorn.

- Up your veg intake: peas, broccoli, carrots, beans, cauliflower, squash and leafy greens are all good.

- Oatcakes, rye crackers and wholegrain rice cakes all make simple snacks, especially topped with pâté, cheese or a vegetable salsa.

- Whenever possible, eat fruit and vegetables in their skin.

- Try dunking carrot, pepper and celery sticks into hummus or other bean dips.

- Add the finishing touch to salads or sandwich fillings with a sprinkling of sprouted grains, beans or lentils.

- Blend cooked split red lentils into curry sauces, soups or stews.

The Benefits of Resistant Starch

The buzzword of the moment in nutrition research is resistant starch. A carbohydrate, best described as a form of dietary fibre, resistant starch is found in a number of foods, including bananas (the more underripe the better), plantains, peas, beans, lentils, wholegrains, potatoes, sweet potatoes, nuts and seeds. Foods containing resistant starch avoid digestion in the small intestine, so move to the colon where they ferment and act like a prebiotic, feeding beneficial gut bacteria and supporting the health of the digestive system. There is a growing body of research to support a wide range of health benefits of resistant starch, including:

- Helps to stabilize blood sugar levels and improve insulin sensitivity, reducing the risk factors of type 2 diabetes and heart disease.
- Ensures sustained energy levels.
- Satisfies the appetite and keeps you full for long periods.
- Encourages you to eat less, leading to weight control and even weight loss.
- Boosts metabolism.
- Improves gut health, helping constipation, IBS, Crohn's disease and other digestive disorders.
- Reduces inflammation in the body, lowering the risk of certain cancers, including bowel.

There are various forms of resistant starch and, interestingly, it is possible to change the amount in a food through the way you prepare and cook it.

Easy ways to increase resistant starch in food:
- Cook wholegrain/black/red rice and then leave it to cool and/or chill. Serve as part of a salad.
- Freeze and defrost bananas to make ice cream (see page 118) or add to a smoothie.
- Leave cooked potatoes or pasta to cool, preferably chill, overnight. Serve in salads or reheat.
- Add lentils or beans to soups, stews and salads.
- Instead of porridge, try overnight oats (see page 46). Soak the oats in milk or water and leave in the fridge overnight. Serve topped with nuts and seeds.
- Freeze and defrost bread.

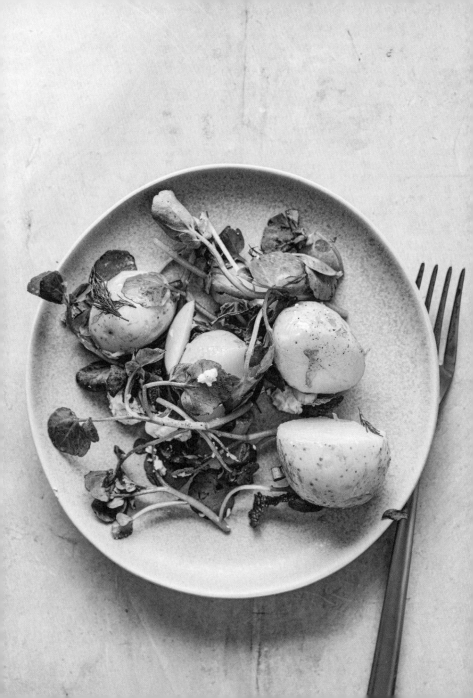

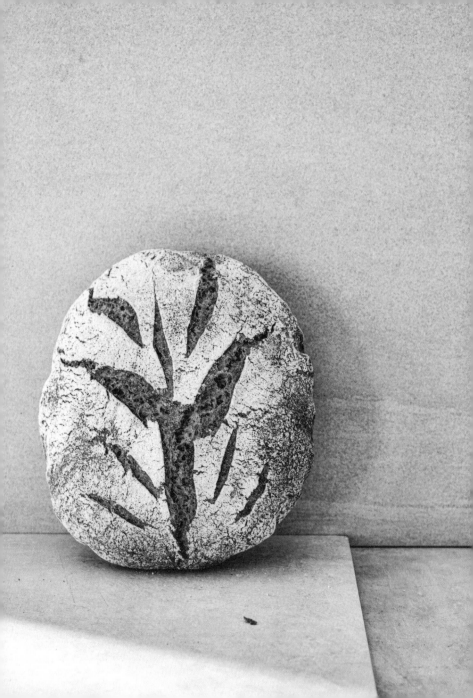

Bread

Much of the criticism of carbs has been levelled at bread, with many people saying they are gluten-intolerant or coeliac. However, there's growing evidence that a sensitivity could be due to new strains of wheat and the methods used in the mass-production of cheap white bread. New strains of wheat are likelier to have higher levels of gluten since this gives a fluffier, more voluminous and consequently higher-yielding loaf. What's more, when the wheat is combined with commercial yeast it creates a quick-rise dough that has been linked to an increase in digestive problems, including intolerance, bloating and discomfort.

Ancient strains of wheat, such as spelt, have been found to be less intrusive on the digestive system, as have traditional forms of breadmaking, such as sourdough. Rather than commercial yeast, sourdough relies on a mix of the lactic acid bacteria in the flour and wild yeasts found naturally in the air to leaven the dough. Since microbes have more time to break down the protein in the flour during the rising/proving stages, many find sourdough easier to digest. Additionally, slow fermentation improves the nutritional profile of sourdough, increasing the bioavailability of the minerals found in wholegrain flour. The absorption of minerals in wholegrains can be limited due to the presence of phytates, yet one study showed that the slow fermentation process may reduce the phytate content by almost half.

Do We Really Need Carbs?

For those who dismiss carbs as surplus to dietary requirements, it's worth considering that this group of foods provides numerous health benefits. For starters, they are our body's main – and preferred – source of energy. They are broken down into glucose in the body, which helps to fuel every cell as well as the brain, heart and nervous system. When glucose levels decrease, mental and physical performance can drop too, leaving us feeling tired and fuzzy-headed. Try to stick to eating the right carbs (see page 10) and cutting down, or cutting out, the wrong ones (see page 13). Here are just a few of the many health benefits of carbs:

Right carbs and heart disease
Carbohydrates are not bad for your heart as long as you eat a good variety of whole, minimally processed carbs in moderate amounts, and avoid refined alternatives. A 10-year Spanish study of 17,424 middle-aged adults found that those eating a proportion of good-quality wholegrains experienced a 47 per cent reduction in the risk of heart disease. Similarly, including moderate recommended amounts of wholegrains (see page 10) in your diet has been found to reduce the risk of stroke.

Right carbs and diabetes
Eating the right type, mix and quantity of carbs is the best way to control blood sugar and prevent type 2 diabetes. High-fibre foods are especially beneficial as they help to keep blood sugar and cholesterol levels under control but do consult your doctor if you are diabetic or have underlying health issues.

Right carbs and exercise
If you exercise regularly, then carbs are your friend, providing much-needed fuel to keep you active. Yet, understanding your optimal carb intake depends on a number of factors: age, sex, activity level, body composition and metabolism. Depending on how often you exercise and the level of intensity, you may need to adjust your carb intake accordingly – even on a daily basis.

It's unnecessary to carb-load before exercising unless you are a planning a high-intensity workout or run that lasts longer than 2 hours. Carb-loading (eating more pasta, bread, potatoes or rice for a period of time prior to an activity) helps to improve endurance and boost performance but, for most of us, it's sufficient to eat a regular diet based on sensible amounts of the right carbs (see page 10). If you're lacking in energy and planning on exercising, then eating a low GI food, such as a slice of wholewheat bread or couple of no-sugar oatcakes, 2–4 hours before exercise may give you the extra oomph you need.

Right carbs and weight control

While the focus of some diets, such as Atkins and South Beach, is on cutting down carbs, eating the right type in moderate amounts can be equally effective in weight control. People who eat moderate amounts of the right carbs have been shown to have a lower body mass index (BMI) and a reduced likelihood of being overweight. Foods high in resistant starch (see page 18) can also play a part as they speed up the metabolism and encourage fat burning, especially around the belly and waist, where storing fat can be particularly harmful, increasing the risk of heart disease, type 2 diabetes and certain cancers.

Finding your optimum amount of carbs is dependent on a number of factors. Those who are physically active and have more muscle mass are able to tolerate more carbs without putting on weight, while those who have a more sedentary lifestyle have a lower tolerance.

Switching to a diet based on high-fibre carbs naturally means less refined and processed foods, so fewer pies, cakes, biscuits and chips. Carbs that are high in fibre fill you up, keep you fuller for longer and subsequently can prevent overeating. In a study published by the American Journal of Clinical Nutrition, wholegrains were found to increase calorie loss as their high-fibre content meant that they passed through the body more quickly than refined alternatives.

Low-carb weight-loss diets are extremely popular, but whether they work or are good for our long-term health is more controversial. People who follow a rigid low-carb diet, or any restrictive diet, often find it difficult to stick to it for any length of time.

Right carbs and a healthy gut

The health of our gut has a major impact on our well-being, both mental and physical. A well-functioning gut features a healthy population of microbes, such as bacteria, fungi and viruses, which not only protect and support our immune system, but reduce the risk of heart disease and diabetes, play a critical role in digestion, release nutrients from food and help weight control.

One of the best ways to improve gut health is to eat more fibre in the form of wholegrains, pulses, nuts, seeds, fruit and vegetables. Fibre supports the good bacteria in the gut, while refined and processed foods work in the opposite way and may even increase levels of harmful bacteria.

Certain carbs, such as chicory, the skin of apples, pulses, onions and Jerusalem artichokes, play a prebiotic role feeding the good strains of bacteria and stimulating their growth, while carbs high in resistant starch also support the health of the gut (see page 18). So, for the best gut health, try to eat as wide and varied a selection of right carbs as possible.

Right carbs and sleep

Studies into the correlation between sleep and diet suggest that eating a right-carb dinner around 4 hours before bedtime can increase sleepiness and reduce the time it takes to fall asleep. If you have difficulty sleeping, eating starchy carbs combined with protein before bedtime may enhance the quality and quantity of your sleep. This is due to the fact that carbohydrates make tryptophan, the amino acid that causes sleepiness, more available to the brain. Tryptophan is found in protein so combining the two food groups is ideal. Sugar, on the other hand, can rob you of sleep. Eating a sugary food too close to bedtime can cause an erratic night's sleep as blood sugar levels rise and fall.

Eat a sleep-enhancing snack 2–3 hours before bedtime to allow time for digestion.

Sleepy food snack combinations:

- Almond butter on wholewheat toast.
- Banana and unsweetened oat milk smoothie.
- Porridge with whole milk.
- Wholegrain seedy crackers with hummus.
- Boiled egg with wholewheat toast.
- Greek-style yogurt with kiwi fruit and nuts.
- Wholegrain cereal with warm milk.
- Cottage cheese with carrot sticks.

Right carbs and mood

A diet high in refined carbs, such as sugary snacks, sweets, drinks and white bread, has not only been linked to weight gain but to an increased risk of depression too. The department of psychiatry at Columbia University Medical Center studied the types of carbohydrate eaten by more than 70,000 post-menopausal women over a four-year period and found that those eating high levels of added sugar and refined carbs had an increased risk of new-onset depression. Women who ate more wholegrains, fruit (not juice), vegetables, dairy and fibre enjoyed a decreased risk of depression. It was found that refined carbs triggered a hormonal response to reduce blood sugar levels, which affected mood and led to fatigue and other symptoms of depression. Researchers concluded that although the study concentrated on post-menopausal women, there is no reason to believe that the results would not apply to men and other age groups as well.

New research also shows that fibre from carbohydrates fuels healthy gut bacteria which may help boost serotonin, the body's feel-good chemical. Carbs may help memory too. A study found that women following a low-carb diet performed worse than those on a low-calorie diet when tested for their cognitive skills, memory and attention span.

Shop & Cook the Right Carb Way

The majority of right carb foods are everyday storecupboard ingredients –
brown rice, wholewheat pasta, beans, peas and lentils – so it pays to stock
up on a good range, then supplement them with fresh fruit and vegetables.
I would also add nuts and seeds to the list, for although they contain fat and
protein, they provide respectable amounts of carbs and fibre. Try to buy the
least processed option possible, as it will be the most nutritious. If your purse
allows, opt for organic to avoid unwanted chemical residues.

Wholegrains

For many of us, grains are our major source of carbs. They are also the focus of
much negativity, and rightly so in some cases. Grains are the seeds of grass-like
plants called cereals, and while we often stick to the familiar wheat and rice,
there are many types, including oats, corn, kamut, barley, freekeh, rye, spelt and
millet. There are also pseudo-cereals (they're actually seeds but are treated as
grains), including quinoa, buckwheat and amaranth.

In their whole form, grains are rich in fibre, vitamins B, E and K, zinc,
iron, magnesium, potassium, antioxidants and plant compounds, such as
polyphenols and sterols.

Refined grains, on the other hand, including white rice, bread, flour and pasta,
have had the germ and bran removed through grinding, flaking and crushing,
which strips or diminishes their nutrients – about 50 per cent of their B
vitamins, 90 per cent of vitamin E and virtually all fibre, although sometimes
these nutrients are added back through fortification. It is believed that the
body cannot distinguish between a teaspoon of sugar and a teaspoon of white
flour in terms of its effect on blood sugar levels.

Cooking grains

The simplest way to cook grains is to put soaked or rinsed grains in a saucepan, cover with water, season with salt and bring to the boil. Reduce the heat to low, cover with a lid, and simmer until the grains are tender; drain, if necessary, and serve. For a flavour and nutrient boost, cook grains in stock or with fresh or canned tomatoes or passata, and with some herbs and/or spices. A splash of extra virgin olive oil or knob of butter stirred in at the end gives extra flavour and a nutritional hit.

Sprouting grains (beans, lentils and seeds)

We are probably most familiar with sprouted beans and lentils, but wholegrains can be sprouted, too. Sprouting makes grains easier to digest by neutralizing phytates and enzyme inhibitors and enhances key nutrients, including B vitamins, folate, vitamin C, iron as well as fibre. Sprouted grains can also be dried and ground into flour to make bread or pastry.

How to sprout

This method is simple to follow and doesn't require any specialist equipment, although a sprouter kit is useful if you're going to be sprouting regularly. Millet, rice, spelt, quinoa, barley, oats, rye, amaranth and corn can all be sprouted. The method is the same for all (as well as beans, lentils and seeds), although the germination time can vary between 1 and 5 days, depending on their size.

- Put 4 tablespoons of wholegrains (or beans, lentils or seeds) in a sieve and rinse under cold running water. Drain well.
- Tip the grains into a large, sterilized jam jar and pour in enough water to cover by 5cm/2 in. Cover the top of the jar with a piece of muslin/cheesecloth and secure with an elastic band. Leave overnight at room temperature and away from direct sunlight.
- The next day, drain the water through the muslin/cheesecloth and re-cover the grains with fresh water. Shake the jar gently, then pour off the water.

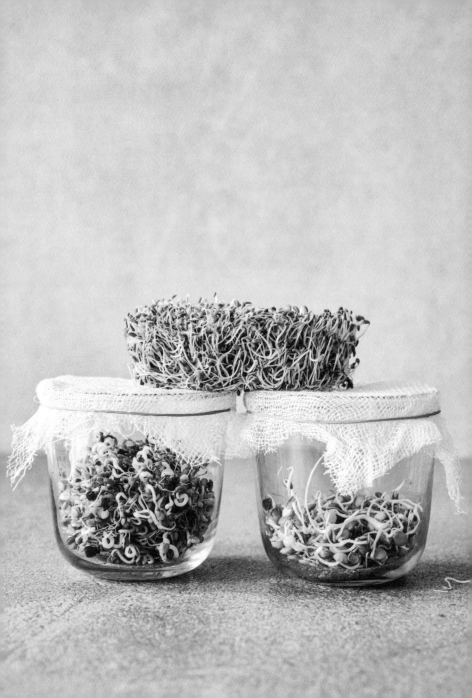

Drain thoroughly and leave the jar on its side and at a slight angle to allow the air to circulate and any residual water to drain away. Place the jar in a draught-free place, away from direct sunlight.

- Rinse and drain thoroughly twice a day until the grains sprout to about 5mm/¼ in. This can take 1–5 days.
- Rinse the sprouts, letting them drain well and removing any grains that haven't germinated. Transfer them to an airtight container and store in the fridge for up to 3 days. Alternatively, dry the sprouted grains in a dehydrator or low oven and grind into a flour.

Store sprouts carefully as recommended above, as they can be a source of bacterial growth, including *E. coli*. Make sure all your equipment and hands are thoroughly clean.

Soaking Grains (Beans, Lentils, Nuts & Seeds)

I haven't specified soaking grains, pulses, nuts or seeds before use in the recipes, but if time allows then this helps to break down the tough outer layer that is difficult to digest as well as increasing the bioavailability of nutrients. Soaking neutralizes the phytates and enzyme inhibitors found in the grains and increases their beneficial enzymes.

How to Soak

- Put your wholegrains in a mixing bowl and pour over twice the volume of warm water – this helps to activate the grain. Stir in 1 tablespoon of plain yogurt or lemon juice and leave to soak overnight at room temperature. The acidity of the yogurt or lemon juice helps the enzymes do their job but isn't completely necessary.

- Drain the grains, rinse well and drain again. The grains can be turned into a 'milk' by blending with 4 parts water or cooked or dried.

Pulses

Pulses – peas, beans and lentils – are one of the most underrated of foods yet are a fantastic addition to the right carb kitchen. They are high in fibre, complex carbohydrates, protein, vitamins and minerals, especially B vitamins, iron, calcium, zinc and potassium, antioxidants and plant compounds. Cheap, versatile and convenient they also count towards the recommended five-a-day (about 3 heaped tablespoons counts as one portion).

For the sake of convenience, I've opted for canned beans and lentils in most of the recipes. Perfect for when you don't have the time to soak or cook dried beans, it's always a good idea to have a few cans to hand. My go-to are chickpeas, kidney beans, butter (lima) beans, black-eyed beans (peas), borlotti, flageolet and cannellini.

If you want to swap the canned beans for dried, follow the instructions on the next page for soaking and cooking. Remember that dried beans double their weight when cooked, so always halve the quantity stated in the recipe if you want to use dried. A standard 400g/14 oz can of chickpeas contains both the chickpeas and liquid or aquafaba (save this to use as an alternative to egg white), so you need to check the drained weight of the beans on the label – roughly 235g/8½ oz chickpeas. Check the label for added sugar, salt or additives too. Some pulses, such as butter (lima) beans, cannellini and lentils, benefit from rinsing first to get rid of any claggy residue.

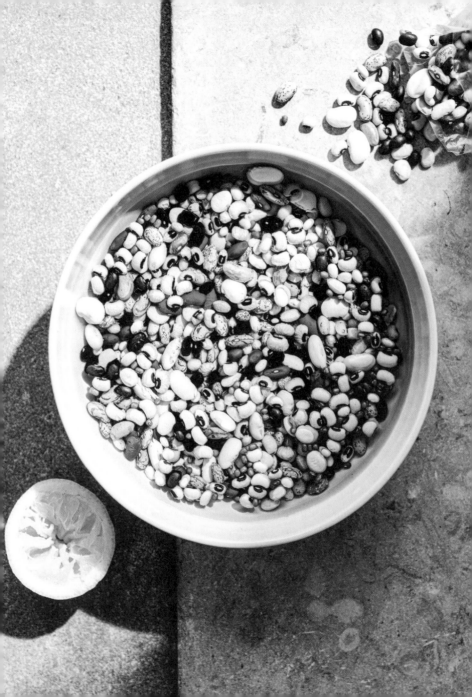

Soaking Pulses

When buying dried beans, look for ones that are smooth, plump and unwrinkled. With a few exceptions, beans benefit from pre-soaking, speeding up cooking time, cooking more evenly and making them more nutritious and easier to digest, with less windy side effects. Mung beans, lentils and split peas don't need to be soaked, but should be rinsed really well until the water runs clear before cooking.

- To soak, rinse the dried beans and pick out any damaged ones. Place in a bowl and cover with about double the volume of water. Leave to soak at room temperature for 6–8 hours or overnight if possible. Drain and rinse before cooking.

- If time is short, try the quick-soak method. Rinse the beans and place in a saucepan. Cover with plenty of cold water and bring to the boil, cook for 2 minutes, then remove from the heat and leave the beans for 1 hour in the hot water. Drain and rinse before cooking.

Cooking Pulses

This is the easiest way to cook pulses. Avoid adding salt during cooking as it can toughen the skin – I prefer to add it to the dish at the end so that I'm not double-salting. Some people recommend adding bicarbonate of soda to speed up cooking and soften the pulses, but this can taint the flavour and turn them mealy in texture. If you are not going to use the cooked pulses straightaway, store them in an airtight container in the fridge for up to 3 days or freeze for up to 3 months.

- Put the peas, beans or lentils, soaked or not, in a saucepan and pour in enough cold water to cover by about 4cm/1½ in. Nutrients leach into the cooking water so you don't want to add too much, and you can always top up when needed.

- Bring to the boil, cover with a lid and boil for 5 minutes (kidney beans need to be boiled for 10 minutes to destroy toxins in the beans). Reduce the heat and simmer the beans, partially covered with a lid, gently stirring occasionally and scooping off any scum that rises to the surface, until tender. Drain and discard the cooking water. Cooking times will vary depending on the type and age of the pulse, ranging from 30 minutes to 3 hours. A pressure cooker reduces the time by about three-quarters.

Sprouting Pulses

Mung bean sprouts are the most popular and readily available sprouts to buy – they're the ones used in Asian cooking – although it is now possible to buy a wider range of sprouts, such as sprouted aduki (adzuki) beans, lentils and chickpeas. Super nutritious, sprouted pulses contain a far higher concentration of vitamins, minerals and protein than their unsprouted counterparts. They are also easier to digest.

It's well worth having a go at sprouting and it's relatively easy to do: aduki (adzuki) beans, chickpeas, whole (not split) lentils and, of course, mung beans are all good for starters. Follow the method for sprouting grains (see page 27) for fresh sprouts that will keep for up to 3 days in the fridge. Remember to sterilize the jar or equipment first and keep everything scrupulously clean to avoid any contamination.

Vegetables

When we think of carbohydrates, vegetables don't immediately spring to mind, or if they do then starchy ones (see right) are the obvious choice. Yet, all vegetables contain carbs to varying degrees, as well as a whole gamut of good things – vitamins, minerals, phytochemicals, antioxidants, fibre and, perhaps surprisingly, some protein. Nutritionally, you can't beat eating a variety of colourful vegetables – starchy and non-starchy. They reduce the risk of many chronic illnesses, including heart disease, cancer, strokes, obesity and high blood pressure.

The big difference between starchy and non-starchy vegetables is their carb content. While some people avoid starchy vegetables, when eaten in sensible amounts they can play a valuable part in good health, especially keeping the digestive system working efficiently. Starchy veg may contain 3–6 times more carbs than non-starchy alternatives, but they do not tend to cause a spike in blood sugar levels (especially if left unpeeled) and this has much to do with their fibre and resistant starch content.

Starchy Vegetables:

- Potatoes
- Sweet potatoes
- Carrots
- Parsnips
- Yams
- Swede (rutabaga)
- Celeriac (celery root)
- Corn
- Pumpkin and squash
- Peas

Non-Starchy Vegetables:

- Leafy greens
- Salad leaves
- Broccoli
- Cauliflower
- Globe artichokes
- Asparagus
- Cabbage
- Mushrooms
- Cucumber
- Tomatoes
- Onions
- Courgette (zucchini)
- Aubergine (eggplant)
- Sweet (bell) peppers

Buying & Cooking Vegetables

Fresh or frozen veg are generally the most nutritious, rather than canned or juiced, which lose valuable nutrients and fibre during processing. Choose bright, shiny-skinned vegetables with no sign of wrinkling or discoloration for the best flavour and nutritional value. Try to buy them in usable amounts on a regular basis, rather than in large quantities, since their nutritional value diminishes when stored for long periods. Opt for loose, seasonal, vegetables rather than those packed in plastic.

Both preparation and cooking can affect a vegetable's nutritional value. Scrub rather than peel vegetables to retain nutrients found in or just below the skin. Preparing vegetables just before cooking or serving is also preferable. The longer cut vegetables are exposed to the air, the greater the loss of nutrients. Even better, cut vegetables up after cooking, if feasible, to prevent water-soluble vitamins leaching into the cooking water.

Steaming, grilling, roasting, baking, stewing and sautéing are preferable to boiling. If you do boil vegetables use a small quantity of water and save it for making stocks or adding to dishes.

Sautéing, stir-frying or shallow-frying vegetables in oil for a short period of time prevents the loss of some nutrients, such as vitamins B and C. Cooking them in oil also enhances the bioavailability of some plant compounds and antioxidants. For instance, beta-carotene, the precursor to vitamin A, was found to be more than six times higher in stir-fried carrots than raw. Similarly, tomatoes have higher levels of the antioxidant lycopene when cooked. That said, it's good to eat a combination of both raw and cooked vegetables – variety is key.

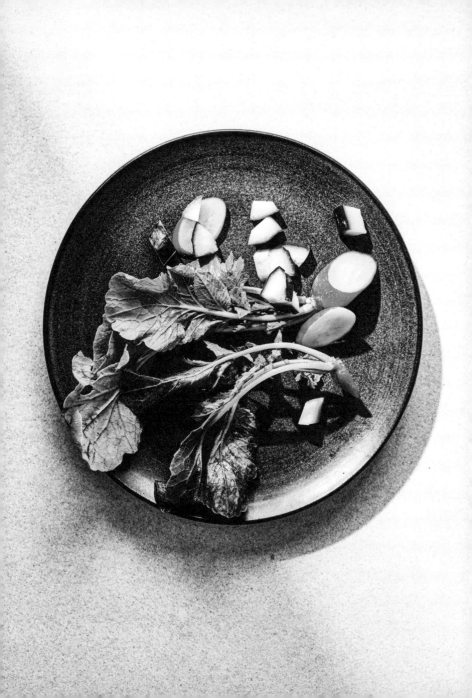

Fruit

A no-no for some advocates of low-carb diets, fruit contains an abundance of nutrients and can play a valuable part in a healthy diet. Many of the nutrients found in fruit – vitamins, minerals, phytochemicals, antioxidants, fibre – are found in or just below the skin so leave them unpeeled whenever possible. The fibre in the skin also slows down the absorption and digestion of the sugars, which explains why it's much better to eat a whole piece of fruit, rather than drink a glass of fruit juice. Eating fruit raw means that you get a higher amount of these vitamins. If you want to opt for low GI fruit, berries, melon, peaches, oranges, cherries and plums are your best options.

When making fruit compotes or stewed fruit, keep the skin on and only use a splash of water to ensure that you retain as much of the water-soluble vitamins – particularly B and C – as possible.

Freezing Fruit & Vegetables

Most fruit and vegetables can be frozen and it's a perfect way to extend their shelf life, especially if you have a glut. Most need a certain amount of prep to ensure they retain their nutritional value, flavour and texture when defrosted. Think about how you like to serve them: chop broccoli into florets, for instance, separating and slicing the stems; grate cauliflower, if you like to serve cauli rice; slice or chop carrots, trim beans; and de-stem leafy greens, for example. Most vegetables benefit from blanching before freezing and it helps keep their colour and texture, although winter squash and tomatoes are exceptions to the rule. Blanch vegetables in salted boiling water for a few minutes until slightly wilted or softened but not cooked, then drain and refresh in a bowl of iced water or under cold running water. Drain well and pat dry with kitchen paper. Lay evenly on a baking sheet lined with baking (parchment) paper and freeze until firm. Once frozen, transfer to a freezer bag and keep for up to 3 months.

If freezing potatoes, leave unpeeled and cut them into the desired size and shape, then blanch until slightly softened and steam dry in a colander or saucepan. Leave to cool before freezing. Pre-cooking and freezing is the perfect way to increase levels of resistant starch (see page 18).

Open-tray freezing is also the best way to freeze fruits such as berries, plums, peaches, grapes, apple and pears. They don't require blanching but do rinse and pat dry beforehand and chop or slice fruit, if needed.

01

Rise 'n' Shine

Mixed Grain Porridge with Cinnamon, Hazelnuts & Apple

Carbs 43.8g
Fibre 7.8g
Calories 408 kcal
per serving

Warming spices such as cinnamon have a natural sweetness that means you don't need to add any extra sugar, especially to dishes such as porridge, fruit compotes and stewed or baked fruit. Rich in polyphenol antioxidants, which play a protective role in the body, cinnamon has been found to help control blood sugar levels – a maximum of 1 teaspoon per person per day is recommended.

Serves 4
Prep: 10 minutes, plus soaking
Cook: 5 minutes

200g/7 oz/1¹/₃ cups mixed flaked grains, such as oats, rye, spelt, quinoa or buckwheat
500ml/17 fl oz/2 cups unsweetened almond milk, or milk of choice
1½ tsp ground cinnamon, plus extra to serve

To serve
4 heaped tbsp Greek-style yogurt
2 red-skinned apples, halved, cored and thinly sliced
50g/1¾ oz/scant ½ cup toasted hazelnuts, roughly chopped
1 tbsp shelled hemp seeds

Put your choice of grains in a pan and pour over 500ml/ 17 fl oz/2 cups water. Leave to soak for at least 30 minutes, or overnight if easier. When you are ready to cook the porridge, pour in the milk, then add the cinnamon and simmer over a medium-low heat for 5 minutes, stirring continuously, until thick and creamy. Add more water or milk, if needed.

Spoon the porridge into serving bowls and top with the yogurt, apple, hazelnuts, hemp seeds and an extra sprinkling of cinnamon.

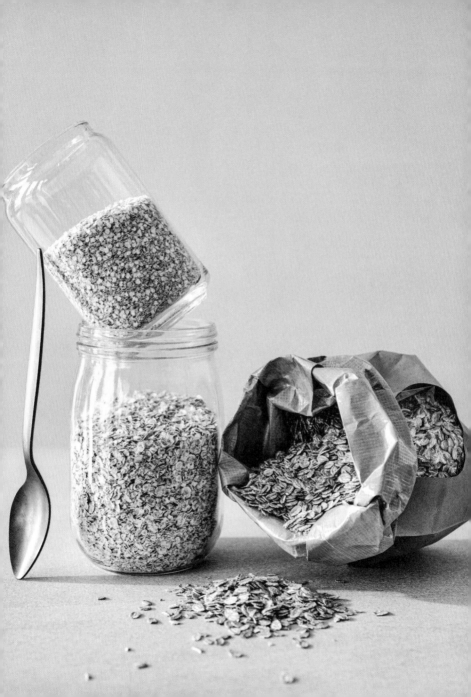

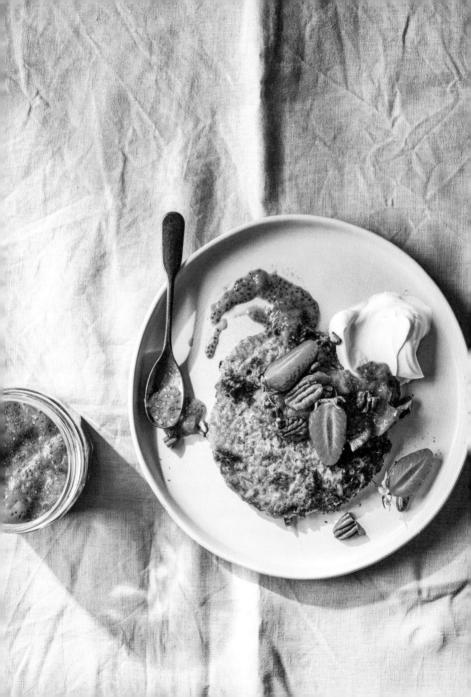

Cottage Cheese Pancakes with Fresh Strawberry Jam

Carbs 24.4g
Fibre 5.2g
Calories 289 kcal
per serving

Cottage cheese ups the protein content of these American-style pancakes, and along with the fibre-rich carbs from the oats they make a satisfying breakfast. The no-added sugar jam relies on the flavour of the fresh strawberries for its sweetness so choose perfectly ripe berries. For a savoury alternative, serve the pancakes topped with a poached egg and grilled tomatoes instead.

Serves 4
Prep: 15 minutes, plus resting
Cook: 20 minutes

115g/4 oz/1^1/$_3$ cups rolled oats
3 large eggs
200g/7 oz/generous ¾ cup cottage cheese
1 tbsp melted butter, plus extra for cooking
pinch of sea salt
1 tsp bicarbonate of soda (baking soda)
Greek-style yogurt and toasted pecans, chopped, to serve

For the fresh strawberry jam
225g/8 oz strawberries, hulled
2 tsp chia seeds
½ tsp vanilla extract
1 tsp lemon juice

First make the fresh strawberry jam. Purée half the strawberries using a stick blender and stir in the chia seeds. Leave for 30 minutes, stirring occasionally, or until the seeds swell and thicken the fruit purée.

Using the back of a fork, roughly mash the rest of the strawberries and stir in the vanilla and lemon juice. Stir the strawberries into the chia mixture and set aside, allowing the jam to thicken further, while you make the pancakes.

To make the pancake batter, blend the oats, eggs, cottage cheese, melted butter, pinch of salt and bicarbonate of soda together to make a smooth, thick batter.

Heat enough butter to lightly coat the base of a large, non-stick frying pan (skillet). Add 3 tablespoons of batter per pancake to the pan – you'll be able to cook 3–4 at a time – and cook for 2–3 minutes on each side until golden. Keep warm in a low oven while you make the rest of the pancakes – the batter makes about 12.

Serve the pancakes with a good spoonful of the jam and some yogurt on the side with pecans scattered over the top.

Overnight Oats with Chia & Berries

Carbs 38.5g
Fibre 10.4g
Calories 648kcal
per serving

My go-to breakfast, these overnight oats are topped with warm milk just before serving to make a satisfying type of 'uncooked' porridge, suped-up with nuts, seeds and cinnamon. A topping of fresh or defrosted frozen fruit adds the finishing touch and just the right level of sweetness. Like other grains, oats are most nutritious and easier to digest after soaking. Rich in a type of fibre called beta-glucan, oats can help improve the health of the gut and enhance the immune system – they also make a great filling start to the day.

Serves 1

Prep: 10 minutes, plus overnight soaking

Cook: 2 minutes

40g/1½ oz/½ cup jumbo oats

½ tbsp chia seeds

250ml/9 fl oz/1 cup plus 2 tbsp full-fat (whole) milk, or milk of choice

1 tbsp toasted sunflower seeds

2 tsp milled flaxseeds

3 walnut halves, roughly broken

2 Brazil nuts, roughly chopped

½ tsp ground cinnamon, plus extra for sprinkling

your choice of fresh or frozen (defrosted) fruit, to serve

Tip the oats and chia seeds into a cereal bowl, pour over 100ml/3½ fl oz/scant ½ cup of the milk, then stir well. Cover and leave in the fridge for at least 1 hour, or overnight if possible.

Remove from the fridge, preferably 30 minutes before serving so the oats have time to come to room temperature, then add the seeds, nuts and cinnamon.

Heat the remaining milk in a small saucepan until hot, then pour it over the oats and stir until combined. Top with your favourite fruit and a sprinkling of cinnamon before serving.

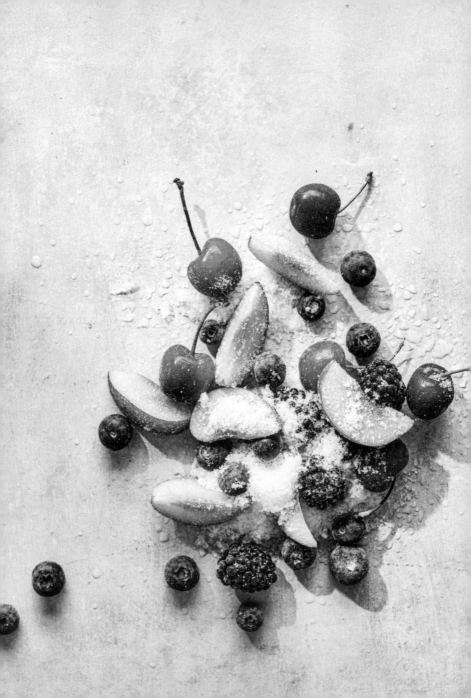

Pasta & Parmesan Pancakes

Carbs 16.5g
Fibre 3.6g
Calories 239 kcal
per serving

These pancakes are a perfect way to use up any leftover cooked spaghetti – wholewheat of course – and they make the perfect fuel for the morning ahead. Cooking pasta and then leaving it to cool increases levels of resistant starch (see page 18), which doesn't appear to be lost if the pasta is subsequently reheated. Resistant starch is a form of fibre, which acts like a prebiotic and generally benefits the health of the gut. Serve the pancakes with grilled vine-ripened tomatoes.

Serves 4
Prep: 10 minutes
Cook: 20 minutes

3 large eggs, lightly beaten
1 tbsp milled flaxseeds
40g/1½ oz/⅓ cup Parmesan cheese, finely grated
250g/9 oz cooked whole wheat spaghetti (about 75g/2½ oz dried weight)
unsalted butter, for cooking
sea salt and black pepper
grilled vine-ripened tomatoes, to serve

Mix together the eggs, flaxseeds and Parmesan in a large mixing bowl. Stir in the cooked spaghetti and season with salt and pepper.

Heat a large frying pan over a high heat, then reduce the heat to medium. Melt enough butter to lightly coat the base of the pan. Add a spoonful of the batter mixture, about 3 tablespoons per pancake, and repeat to cook 2–3 pancakes at a time. Cook for 2 minutes on each side or until set and light golden. Repeat to make about 8 pancakes in total. Serve the pancakes with grilled tomatoes on the side.

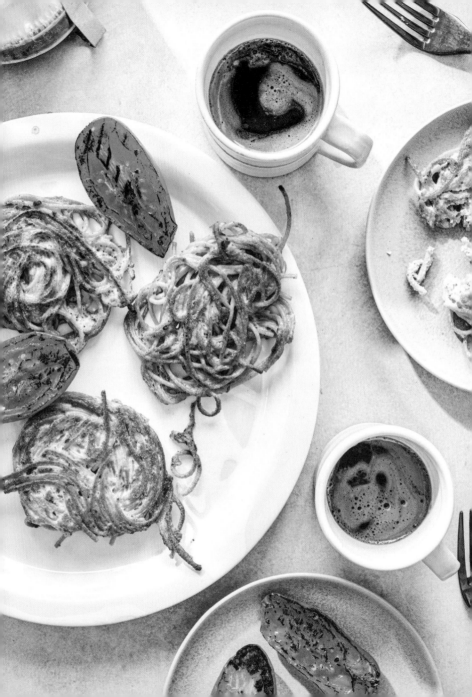

Smoky Mushrooms & Beans

Carbs 16.0g
Fibre 6.8g
Calories 168 kcal
per serving

Shop-bought baked beans more often than not contain added sugar and/or artificial sweetener, neither of which is necessary. This borlotti bean version has a delicious smoky flavour from the chipotle chilli and comes with the added bonus of vitamin D-rich mushrooms and a creamy protein-boost from the hummus.

Serves 4
Prep: 10 minutes
Cook: 30 minutes

2 tbsp extra virgin olive oil

1 onion, finely chopped

350g/12 oz/6$^1/_3$ cups chestnut (cremini) mushrooms, torn into chunks

2 garlic cloves, finely chopped

1–2 tsp ground chipotle chilli (or dried flakes)

1 tsp dried thyme

400g/14 oz can borlotti beans, drained

400g/14 oz can chopped tomatoes

1 tbsp tomato purée (tomato paste)

2 tsp Worcestershire sauce

1 tsp Dijon mustard

sea salt and black pepper

wholemeal seeded toast and hummus, to serve

Heat a large, deep sauté pan over a medium heat. Add the oil and onion and cook for 5 minutes until softened. Add the mushrooms and cook for a further 8 minutes, adding a splash more oil, if needed. Stir in the garlic, chipotle and thyme and cook for a further minute.

Add the beans, tomatoes, purée, Worcestershire sauce, mustard and 100ml/3½ fl oz/7 tbsp water, stir and bring to a gentle bubble. Reduce the heat slightly and simmer for 15 minutes, partially covered, until reduced and thickened. Season with salt and pepper to taste. Serve with toast and topped with a spoonful of hummus.

Cauliflower & Basmati Kedgeree with Trout

Carbs 34.2g
Fibre 4.2g
Calories 468 kcal
per serving

Grated cauliflower adds both interest and flavour to this rice dish – it's also the perfect addition if you're mindful of overloading on starchy carbs, yet still want a decent-sized serving. If you're looking to serve the kedgeree as a main meal, simply up the veg count with peas, broccoli, spinach or other leafy greens, such as cabbage or chard.

Serves 4

Prep: 20 minutes

Cook: 20 minutes

150g/5½ oz/¾ cup brown basmati rice, rinsed well

1 tsp ground turmeric

40g/1½ oz/3 tbsp butter, ghee or extra virgin coconut oil

1 onion, finely chopped

200g/7 oz cauliflower, grated

100g/3½ oz Savoy cabbage, shredded

1 tsp cumin seeds

2.5cm/1 in piece cinnamon stick

2 garlic cloves, finely chopped

4cm/1½ in piece fresh ginger, peeled and finely chopped

1 green medium-hot chilli, finely chopped

4 hot-smoked pink trout fillets, skin removed, flesh flaked

good squeeze of lemon juice

sea salt and black pepper

Put the rice in a saucepan and pour over enough water to cover by 1cm/½ in. Bring to the boil over a medium-high heat, then stir in the turmeric. Reduce the heat to its lowest setting, cover with a lid and simmer for 20 minutes, or until the grains are tender and the water has been absorbed.

While the rice is cooking, melt the butter in a large, deep sauté pan over a medium-low heat. Add the onion and cook, covered, for 10 minutes until softened but not coloured. Add the cauliflower, cabbage, cumin seeds, cinnamon, garlic and ginger and cook, stirring, for a further 5 minutes until softened. Set aside.

When the rice is ready, stir it into the onion mixture with the chilli and trout. Season with salt and pepper, bearing in mind that the fish is quite salty, then cover and leave to sit for 5 minutes to allow the fish to warm through. Just before serving add a good squeeze of lemon juice.

Savoury Buckwheat Porridge with Mushrooms

Carbs 46.5g
Fibre 8.2g
Calories 489 kcal
per serving

Pure comfort food in a bowl, this warming cheesy buckwheat porridge is topped with fried mushrooms and a poached egg. As well as providing a wide range of vitamins and minerals, buckwheat is a good source of the plant compound rutin, which has been found to support blood sugar control and heart health.

Serves 4
Prep: 10 minutes, plus soaking
Cook: 15 minutes

300g/10½ oz buckwheat groats
1½ tsp vegetable bouillon powder
55g/2 oz/4 tbsp unsalted butter
40 g/1½ oz/⅓ cup mature Cheddar cheese, grated
350g/12 chestnut (cremini) 350g/12 oz/6⅓ cups chestnut (cremini) mushrooms, sliced
4 eggs
2 tbsp snipped chives
sea salt and black pepper

Put the buckwheat in a bowl, pour over enough water to generously cover and leave to soak for 1 hour, or overnight if possible.

To cook the porridge, drain and rinse the buckwheat then tip into a saucepan with 875ml/30 fl oz/3¾ cups water. Bring to the boil and stir in the bouillon powder. Reduce the heat to low and simmer, partially covered with a lid and stirring every so often, for 12–15 minutes until the grains are tender and most of the water has been absorbed – it should be still slightly runny. Stir in 15g/½ oz of the butter and the cheese. Season with pepper.

While the buckwheat is cooking, melt the rest of the butter in a large, deep sauté pan over a medium heat. Add the mushrooms and fry for 8 minutes, turning occasionally, until starting to turn golden. Tip the mushrooms into a bowl and keep warm in a low oven.

Wipe the pan clean and three-quarters fill with just-boiled water from a kettle. Swirl the water clockwise and crack in the eggs, one by one, and poach for 3–4 minutes or until the whites are set but the yolks remain runny. Remove with a slotted spoon and drain on kitchen paper.

Spoon the buckwheat porridge into four large shallow bowls and top with the mushrooms and egg. Season with salt and pepper and scatter over the chives.

Avocado & Miso Butter on Toast

Carbs 23.5g
Fibre 4.8g
Calories 272 kcal
per serving

There's a synergy between good gut health and our overall physical and mental well-being – the gut has even been called our 'second brain'. This nutritious breakfast is an excellent way to support our digestive system at the start of the day. The fibre found in the rye bread helps to increase levels of beneficial bacteria in the gut, while the miso, being fermented, boasts similar properties.

Serves 4
Prep: 10 minutes
Cook: 5 minutes

1 avocado, halved and stoned

2 spring onions (scallions), roughly chopped

25g/1 oz baby spinach leaves

1 large garlic clove, roughly chopped

1 green jalapeño chilli, deseeded and roughly chopped

juice of 1 lime

2 tsp white miso

sea salt and black pepper

Scoop the avocado out of its skin with a spoon and put in a mini blender with the rest of the ingredients. Blend until smooth, then season with pepper. Taste and add a little salt if needed, but as the miso is salty you shouldn't need it. Set aside while you prepare the rye bread and toppings.

Lightly toast the rye bread and, while still warm, top each slice with a generous amount of the avocado mixture. Finish with a grinding of black pepper.

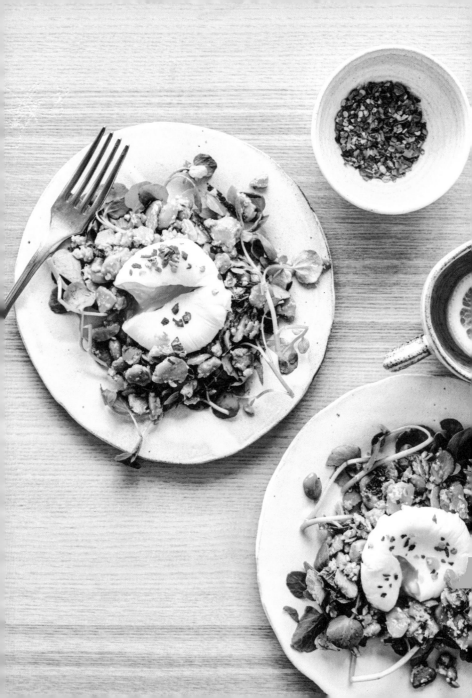

Poached Eggs with Smashed Broad Beans

Carbs 7.7g
Fibre 8.9g
Calories 286 kcal
per serving

You can't go wrong with a bag of broad beans in the freezer. This versatile vegetable makes a nutritious base for poached eggs instead of the more usual toast, and is a winning combination of protein, carbs and fibre as well as providing a fair smattering of B vitamins. Perfect for when fresh beans are out of season, frozen ones make a great hummus or can be added to soups, stews, salads, sauces and stir-fries.

Serves 4
Prep: 15 minutes
Cook: 5 minutes

400g/14 oz/3½ cups frozen (or fresh) podded broad (fava) beans, defrosted if frozen

2 garlic cloves, finely chopped

finely grated zest and juice of 1 unwaxed lemon

4 tbsp extra virgin olive oil

20g/¾ oz/scant ¼ cup Parmesan cheese, finely grated

2 tbsp finely chopped fresh mint

4 large eggs

splash of white wine vinegar

4 large handfuls watercress, tough stalks removed

dried chilli flakes, for sprinkling (optional)

sea salt and black pepper

Steam the broad beans for 3–4 minutes until tender, then leave to cool slightly and pop them out of their grey outer skin to reveal the bright green bean inside. Put the cooked beans in a bowl with the garlic, lemon zest and juice, olive oil and 2 tablespoons of hot water. Mash with the back of a fork until the beans are roughly crushed – if the mixture looks too dry, add a splash more water. Stir in the Parmesan and mint and season with salt and pepper.

Meanwhile, poach the eggs. Bring a large sauté pan three-quarters full of water to the boil, then reduce the heat to low so the water is barely bubbling. Add a splash of vinegar and swirl the water around with a spoon. Crack the eggs into the pan one at a time and poach for 3–4 minutes or until the white is just set – you may need to do this in two batches. Place the cooked eggs on kitchen paper to drain briefly.

To serve, divide the watercress between four plates and top with the smashed broad beans. Using a slotted spoon, scoop the eggs on to the beans. Sprinkle with a few chilli flakes, if using, and season.

02

Small
Plates

Asian Broth with Prawns & Black Bean Noodles

Carbs 11.3g
Fibre 13.1g
Calories 280 kcal
per serving

Not only do black bean noodles look stunning in contrast to the golden broth, green vegetables, pink prawns (shrimp) and red chilli, they come with nutritional benefits. Higher in protein than refined wheat-based noodles, they are also a good source of complex carbs and fibre. Find the noodles in large supermarkets or health food shops. Also, keep an eye out for soya bean or edamame bean noodles, which provide similar health benefits.

Serves 4
Prep: 20 minutes, plus infusing
Cook: 20 minutes

1.2 litres/40fl oz/5 cups chicken or vegetable stock

5 cardamom pods, lightly crushed

2 star anise

8cm/3¼ in piece fresh ginger, peeled and sliced into rounds

200g/7 oz black bean noodles or spaghetti

2 tsp toasted sesame oil

1 tsp ground turmeric

1 red chilli, thinly sliced

1 small red (bell) pepper, deseeded and thinly sliced

6 spring onions (scallions), green and white parts separated, thinly sliced diagonally

250g/9 oz raw king prawns (jumbo shrimp), peeled

55 g/2 oz sugar snap peas

2 handfuls beansprouts

sea salt and black pepper

Put the stock, cardamom, star anise and ginger in a large saucepan and bring to the boil, then reduce the heat and simmer, partially covered with a lid, for 5 minutes. Turn off the heat and leave to infuse for 30 minutes.

Meanwhile, cook the noodles following the packet instructions, then drain and refresh under cold running water. Leave the noodles to sit in cold water.

Just before serving, strain the broth, discarding the aromatics, then return it to the pan and bring to the boil. Reduce the heat and stir in the sesame oil, turmeric, chilli, red pepper and whites of the spring onions and simmer for 2 minutes. Season with salt and pepper to taste.

Add the prawns and sugar snaps and simmer for a further 2–3 minutes until the prawns are cooked through and pink.

Drain the noodles, pour over just-boiled water from a kettle to reheat them, then divide between four large shallow bowls. Ladle the broth over and top with a pile of beansprouts and the green part of the spring onions.

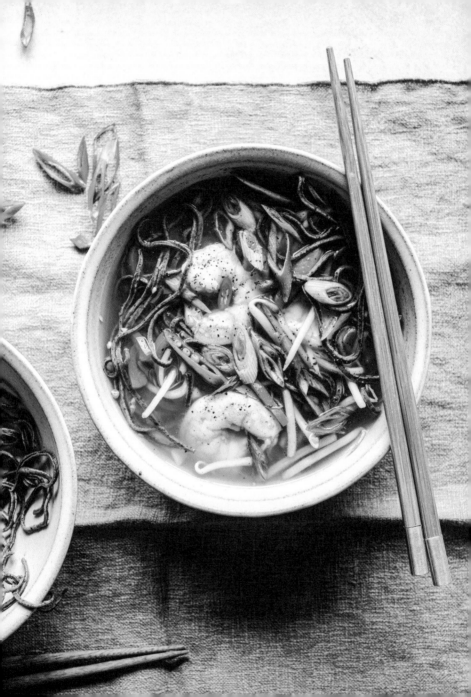

Cannellini Bean Dip with Roasted Red Pepper

Carbs 10.4g
Fibre 4.9g
Calories 114 kcal
per serving

Canned beans are a godsend in the right carb kitchen. Convenient, economical and an excellent source of fibre, plant protein and slow-release carbs, they also count towards your 5-a-day. They are a good source of iron, the absorption of which is enhanced here by the vitamin C in the red pepper.

Serves about 8
Prep: 10 minutes
Cook: 25 minutes

2 red (bell) peppers, deseeded, each cut into 6 wedges

4 large garlic cloves

3 tbsp extra virgin olive oil, plus extra for roasting and drizzling

2 x 400g/14 oz cans cannellini beans, drained and rinsed

finely grated zest of 1 and juice of 2 unwaxed lemons

hot smoked paprika, for sprinkling

sea salt and black pepper

wholemeal (wholewheat) pitta breads and vegetable sticks, such as carrots, long-stem broccoli, sugar snap peas, celery and cucumber, to serve

Preheat the oven to 180°C fan/200°C/400°F/gas mark 6.

Toss the peppers and three of the garlic cloves in oil and spread out on a baking tray (sheet). Roast for 20–25 minutes, turning halfway through cooking, until starting to blacken in places. Remove from the oven, place in a bowl, cover and set aside for 5 minutes – this will make the peppers easier to peel. When cool enough to handle, peel the skins off the peppers and cut them into thin strips.

Squeeze the roasted garlic out of their papery skins and put them in a blender with the remaining raw garlic clove, the beans, lemon juice, lemon zest and 3 tablespoons of olive oil, then blend until smooth and creamy. Season well with salt and pepper.

Spoon the dip into a bowl and top with the red pepper, an extra swirl of oil and a sprinkling of smoked paprika. Serve with pitta breads and vegetable sticks for dipping.

Middle Eastern Spinach & Lentil Soup

Carbs 21.3g
Fibre 8.2g
Calories 266 kcal
per serving

A bowl of this hearty, filling soup with fragrant spices and a hint of lemon provides a healthy combination of complex carbs, protein and fibre as well as an abundance of vitamins and minerals. Brown lentils hold their shape when cooked, although they have a more yielding texture than perhaps Puy or green ones, so work well in a soup or stew.

Serves 4

Prep: 20 minutes

Cook: 35 minutes

2 tbsp extra virgin olive oil

1 large onion, roughly chopped

2 carrots, cut into large dice

1 large celery stick, thinly sliced

2 large garlic cloves, thinly sliced

½ tsp dried chilli flakes

1 tsp cumin seeds

1 tsp coriander seeds, crushed

2 bay leaves

100g/3½ oz/½–⅔ cup brown lentils, rinsed well

2 tbsp tomato purée (tomato paste)

1.4 litres/2½ pints/6 cups vegetable or chicken stock

2 tsp ground paprika

100g/3½ oz baby spinach leaves

juice of ½ lemon

sea salt and black pepper

100g/3½ oz/½ cup Greek-style yogurt, to serve

Heat a large saucepan over a medium heat. Add the oil and onion and cook for 5 minutes until softened, then stir in the carrots, celery, garlic, chilli flakes, cumin and coriander seeds and bay leaves. Reduce the heat slightly and cook for a further 2 minutes, stirring frequently.

Stir in the lentils and tomato purée, then add the stock. Bring to the boil, then reduce the heat to medium-low and simmer, partially covered, for 25 minutes or until the lentils are tender.

Stir in the paprika and spinach and cook for 2 minutes until the leaves have wilted. Just before serving, stir in the lemon juice and season with salt and pepper. Serve topped with a good spoonful of yogurt.

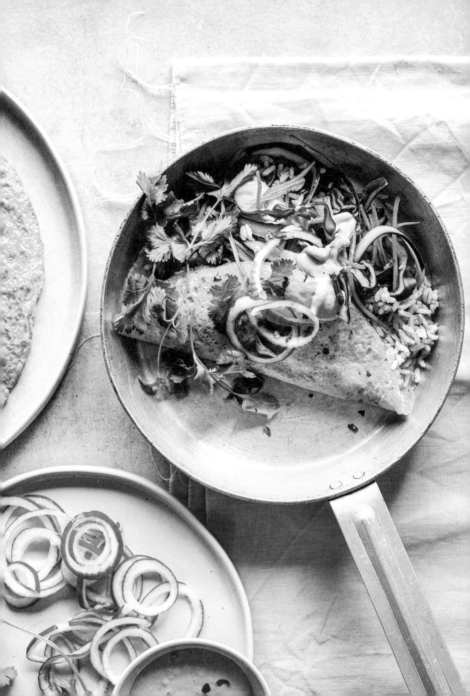

Omelette Wrap with Satay Sauce

Carbs 40.5g
Fibre 6.9g
Calories 668 kcal
per serving

Ring the changes with an omelette wrap, which takes the place of the more usual wheat-based tortilla wrap. The right-carb element comes in the form of brown jasmine rice, which is combined with crunchy raw vegetables, a peanut sauce, lots of herbs and a lively red onion pickle to make a nutritious filling.

Serves 4
Prep: 20 minutes
Cook: 35 minutes

165g/5¾ oz/generous ¾ cup brown jasmine rice, rinsed
1 tbsp toasted sesame seeds
1 small red onion, thinly sliced
2 tbsp raw apple cider vinegar
100g/3½ oz red cabbage, shredded
2 carrots, cut into thin matchsticks
½ cucumber, deseeded and cut into ribbons
1 large handful coriander (cilantro) leaves
8 eggs
40g/1½ oz/3 tbsp butter
sea salt and black pepper

For the satay sauce
150g/5½ oz/²/₃ cup peanut butter
juice of 1 lime
2 tsp light soy sauce
2 tsp toasted sesame oil, plus extra for the salad
5cm/2 in piece fresh ginger, peeled and finely grated
1 large garlic clove, finely grated
½ tsp dried chilli flakes, plus extra to serve

Cook the rice following the packet instructions and drain if needed. Leave to sit for 5 minutes, then stir in the sesame seeds.

Meanwhile, put the onion in a bowl and pour over the vinegar. Set aside to pickle until ready to serve.

Blend together all the ingredients for the satay sauce with 4 tablespoons of just-boiled water in a blender.

Put the cabbage, carrots and cucumber in a bowl, drizzle over a little sesame oil, season with salt and pepper and toss until combined.

To make the omelettes, beat 2 eggs in a bowl and season. Heat a quarter of the butter in a medium frying pan (skillet) over a medium-low heat and add the beaten eggs. Tip the pan to coat the base with the eggs and cook for a minute or two until set. Keep the omelette warm, covered, in a low oven, while you make the remaining three omelettes.

To serve, top the omelettes with the rice and vegetable salad. Spoon over the satay sauce and finish with the onion pickle, coriander and an extra sprinkling of chilli flakes. Serve flat or fold the omelette over to encase the filling.

Chickpea Flour Pizzas

Carbs 46.7g
Fibre 10.8g
Calories 594 kcal
per serving

Chickpea flour – also known as gram or besan flour – makes a great-tasting base for pizzas in place of the more usual wheat flour. Plus, it provides an impressive range of macro- and micro-nutrients – think complex carbs, protein, fibre, iron, magnesium, folate and manganese – and since it contains about half the amount of carbs of refined wheat flour, it doesn't cause a spike in blood sugar levels. What's not to like?

Makes 4

Prep: 20 minutes, plus resting

Cook: 35 minutes

300g/10½ oz/scant 2½ cups chickpea (gram) flour

¾ tsp sea salt

4 tbsp extra virgin olive oil, plus extra for cooking pizzas

200g/7 oz passata (sieved tomatoes)

2 tsp hot smoked paprika

2 tbsp tomato purée (tomato paste)

1 tsp dried oregano

1 red onion, thinly sliced into rounds

4 chestnut (cremini) mushrooms, thinly sliced

250g/9 oz/scant 2¼ cups mozzarella, drained and torn into pieces

1 handful stoned Kalamata olives

4 handfuls rocket leaves

sea salt and black pepper

To make the pizza base, mix together the chickpea flour and salt in a large mixing bowl. Make a well in the centre and pour in 300ml/10½ fl oz/scant 1¼ cups water and the olive oil. Stir with a wooden spoon, gradually drawing the flour into the wet ingredients to make a smooth, thick batter. Leave to rest for at least 30 minutes.

When ready to assemble the pizzas, mix together the passata, paprika, tomato purée and oregano.

Preheat the grill to high.

Heat a medium ovenproof frying pan (skillet) over a medium-high heat. Add 2 teaspoons of olive oil and tilt the pan to coat the base. Pour in a quarter of the batter and spread out with the back of a spoon. Cook for 3–4 minutes until the base is golden and set – the top should be just cooked. Spread a quarter of the tomato sauce on top. Scatter over a quarter of the red onion, mushrooms, mozzarella and olives. Add a drizzle of oil, season with salt and pepper, and place under the hot grill for 3–4 minutes or until the mozzarella has melted and is starting to colour.

Remove from the grill and just before serving top each pizza with a handful of rocket. Repeat to make four pizzas in total.

Buckwheat Pancakes with Creamy Mushrooms

Carbs 42.5g
Fibre 10.3g
Calories 572 kcal
per serving

Buckwheat flour has a slightly more pronounced nutty flavour than wheat flour, making it perfect for both sweet and savoury pancakes, blinis and French-style galettes. It has a lot going for it – a complete protein, meaning it contains all nine essential amino acids, buckwheat is also rich in fibre, B vitamins, magnesium, iron, zinc and selenium.

Serves 4

Prep: 20 minutes, plus resting

Cook: 35 minutes

200g/7 oz/1¼ cups buckwheat flour

½ tsp sea salt

2 eggs

230ml/7¾ fl oz/scant 1 cup whole milk or milk of your choice

For the creamy mushrooms

25g/1 oz/2 tbsp unsalted butter, plus extra for cooking

2 tbsp extra virgin olive oil

400g/14 oz/7 cups chestnut (cremini) mushrooms, thinly sliced

400g/14 oz can cannellini beans, drained and rinsed

300g/10½ oz baby leaf spinach

juice of ½ lemon

5 tbsp crème fraîche or dairy-free alternative

2 tsp Dijon mustard

sea salt and black pepper

To make the pancake batter, mix together the flour and salt in a large mixing bowl and make a well in the middle. Whisk the eggs into the milk with 200ml/7 fl oz/scant 1 cup water until combined. Gradually, pour the egg mixture into well in the flour, stirring with a balloon whisk to make a smooth batter the consistency of thick single (light) cream. Leave to rest for 30 minutes.

While the batter is resting, prepare the creamy mushrooms. Heat a large sauté pan over a medium heat, add the butter and oil and when hot stir in the mushrooms. Fry for 8 minutes, stirring often, until starting to turn golden, then add the beans and spinach. Cook, turning the spinach with tongs, for 3 minutes until wilted. Add the lemon juice, crème fraîche and mustard and warm through for a further couple of minutes. Season with salt and pepper and set aside until ready to serve.

To cook the pancakes, heat a large frying pan until very hot, then reduce the heat to medium. Melt enough butter to very lightly coat the base of the pan and ladle a spoonful of the batter into the pan, tilting it to move the mixture around in an even layer. Cook for 2–3 minutes, turning halfway, or until golden. Keep warm in a low oven while you make the remaining pancakes; the batter should make 8–10 in total.

When ready to serve, gently reheat the creamy mushrooms. Fold the pancakes in half and serve two per person. Top the pancakes with the mushrooms and serve.

Black Beans with Roasted Tomato Salsa

Carbs 40.7g
Fibre 8.7g
Calories 449 kcal
per serving

This recipe is a vibrant combination of fresh vegetables, beans, herbs and feta. In true Tex-Mex style, the various components of this meat-free dish can be laid out for everyone to help themselves or can be assembled before serving. Not only is it sure to revive tired taste buds, this light meal is loaded with plant-based goodness – vitamins, minerals, antioxidants and phytochemicals, not forgetting good carbs.

Serves 4
Prep: 20 minutes
Cook: 15 minutes

1 large avocado, halved, stoned and sliced
juice of 1 large lime
2 courgettes (zucchini), coarsely grated
10 radishes, thinly sliced
1½ tbsp diced red onion
400g/14 oz can black beans, drained and rinsed
2 tbsp extra virgin olive oil
4 small corn tortillas
1 large handful coriander (cilantro) leaves
100g/3½ oz/scant ½ cup feta cheese, crumbled
sea salt and black pepper

For the roasted tomato salsa
300g/10½ oz vine-ripened tomatoes
1 red jalapeño chilli
¾ red onion, cut into wedges
1 garlic clove, peeled
1½ tsp red wine vinegar
½ tsp dried chipotle chilli flakes

First make the roasted tomato salsa. Put the tomatoes in a large, dry frying pan (skillet) over a high heat, turning occasionally, for 5 minutes or until charred in places. Remove from the pan and repeat with the chilli, onion wedges and garlic, turning them occasionally until charred in places.

Put the chilli, onion and garlic in a mini food processor and pulse until roughly chopped. Add the tomatoes and the rest of the salsa ingredients and pulse briefly to make a coarse-textured salsa. Season with salt and pepper and set aside.

Toss the avocado in a little lime juice to stop it from discolouring. Put it in a bowl with the courgettes, radishes, diced onion and black beans. Pour over the olive oil and the rest of the lime juice, season with salt and pepper, then mix gently until combined.

Heat the corn tortillas in the frying pan, one at a time, until crisp. Place on a plate and top with the black bean mixture, tomato salsa, coriander leaves and feta.

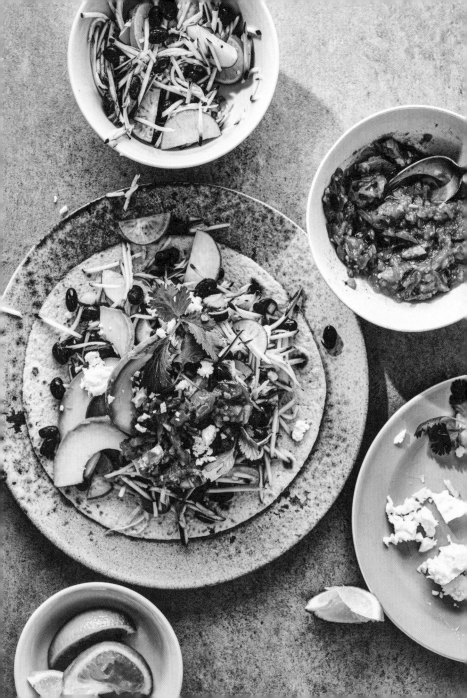

Chilled Soba Noodle Salad with Edamame & Sesame Dressing

Carbs 39.3g
Fibre 10.3g
Calories 358 kcal
per serving

Look for soba noodles that are pure buckwheat, rather than those that also contain refined wheat. Nutritionally, buckwheat is higher in plant-based protein than wheat and is gluten free. Eating the noodles cold means they are higher in resistant starch (see page 18), which helps to improve the health of the gut as well as keep blood sugar levels on an even keel.

Serves 4

Prep: 15 minutes

Cook: 5 minutes

200g/7 oz 100% buckwheat soba noodles

100g/3½ oz/scant 1 cup frozen edamame beans

100g/3½ oz sugar snap peas, sliced diagonally

5 spring onions (scallions), halved diagonally

8 radishes, thinly sliced

½ cucumber, quartered, deseeded and diced

1 tbsp sesame seeds, toasted

2 tbsp nori or dulse flakes (optional)

½ tsp shichimi togarashi (Japanese 7 spice blend)

sea salt and black pepper

For the sesame dressing

3 tbsp toasted sesame oil

2 tbsp light soy sauce

4cm/1½ in piece fresh ginger, peeled and finely grated

Cook the noodles following the packet instructions, usually about 3 minutes. Drain the noodles – in Japan it is customary to drink the cooking water as it contains B vitamins – and refresh under cold running water. Put the noodles in a bowl of cold water and set aside.

Meanwhile, steam the edamame beans until tender, then refresh under cold running water.

Mix together all the ingredients for the dressing. Season with pepper and taste for salt, it may not need any as the soy is quite salty.

To assemble the salad, drain the noodles and put them in a large serving bowl with the edamame, sugar snaps, most of the spring onions, the radishes and cucumber. Pour over the dressing and toss gently until combined. Top with the sesame seeds, nori or dulse, if using, the remaining spring onions and the shichimi togarashi.

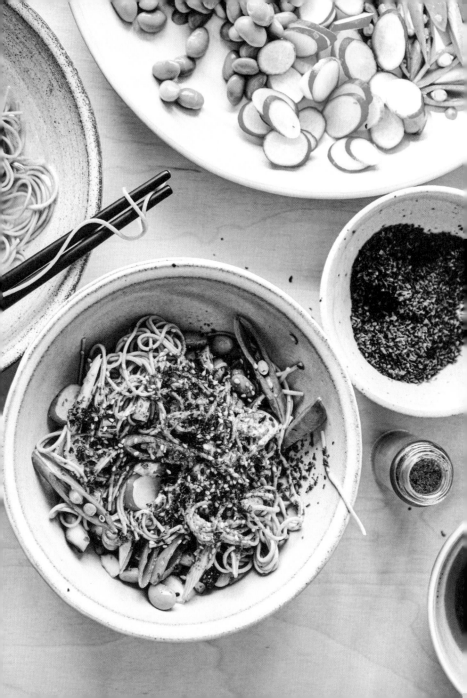

Red Rice & Chicken Salad with Herb Yogurt Dressing

Carbs 22.6g
Fibre 2.8g
Calories 329 kcal
per serving

Dusky red Camargue rice not only looks good, it has been found to be lower in carbs and higher in protein and fibre than both white and, more impressively, brown alternatives. It also provides a healthy dose of antioxidants, especially protective anthocyanins, which are anti-inflammatory and antibacterial. Serve the rice cooled to room temperature to increase the levels of gut-friendly resistant starch (see page 18). This main-meal salad makes the most of leftover roast chicken and comes with an abundance of veg and a light minty yogurt dressing.

Serves 4

Prep: 20 minutes

Cook: 25 minutes

100g/3½ oz/½ cup red rice (or a mixture of red and wild rice), rinsed

100g/3½ oz mixed watercress, spinach and rocket (arugula) leaves

75g/2½ oz sugar snap peas, halved diagonally

3 spring onions (scallions), thinly sliced diagonally

2 celery sticks, thinly sliced

300g/10½ oz leftover roast chicken, torn into strips

extra virgin olive oil, for drizzling

For the herb yogurt dressing

125g/4½ oz/scant ²/₃ cup Greek-style yogurt

1 large handful mint, plus extra to serve

1 large handful flat-leaf parsley, plus extra to serve

juice of ½ lemon

2 spring onions (scallions), chopped

sea salt and black pepper

Cook the rice following the packet instructions until tender, but not mushy. Drain if needed and leave in the strainer to cool while you prepare the rest of the salad.

Blend together all the ingredients for the dressing. Season with salt and pepper. Taste and add more lemon juice if needed.

To assemble the salad, place the salad leaves on a large serving plate and top with the rice, sugar snaps, spring onions, celery and chicken. Pour over enough of the dressing to lightly coat. At this point, you can either toss the salad or serve it in layers. Top with extra mint and parsley leaves and more dressing, if needed.

Black Rice Salad with Tahini Dressing

Carbs 50g
Fibre 9.3g
Calories 493 kcal
per serving

The chewy, nutty texture of black rice works well with the crunch of the vegetables and creaminess of the tahini dressing and it looks dramatic in contrast to the red cabbage, carrots and broccoli. It's also good for you – research shows that black rice is loaded with heart-friendly antioxidants.

Serves 4

Prep: 15 minutes

Cook: 20 minutes

225g/8 oz/generous 1 cup black rice, rinsed well

200g/7 oz long-stem broccoli, stalks trimmed

2 carrots, shredded

140g/5 oz red cabbage, shredded

4 spring onions (scallions), thinly sliced diagonally

2 handfuls coriander (cilantro) leaves

75g/2½ oz/⅔ cup toasted cashews, roughly chopped

For the tahini dressing

3 tbsp tahini

1½ tbsp toasted sesame oil

juice of 1 large lime

1 garlic clove, crushed

2 tsp finely grated fresh ginger

sea salt and black pepper

Cook the rice following the packet instructions until tender. Drain and leave to cool slightly while you prepare the rest of the salad. (The rice can either be served slightly warm or at room temperature.)

Meanwhile, blend together all the ingredients for the dressing, adding 2 tablespoons of water until smooth and creamy. Season well with salt and pepper.

Steam the broccoli for 3 minutes or until just tender, then refresh under cold running water. Slice the stems diagonally and tear the florets if large.

Put the rice in a large serving dish and add the carrots, cabbage, spring onions, broccoli and half the coriander. Toss gently until combined. Scatter the rest of the coriander and cashews over the salad. Put the dressing in a separate bowl and let everyone help themselves, drizzling it over the top just before eating.

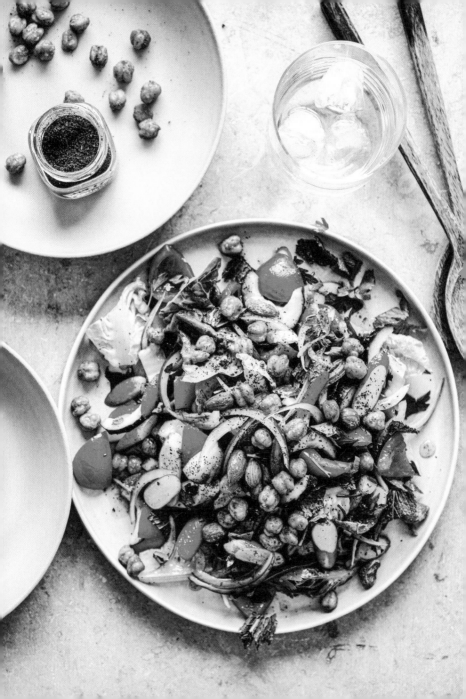

Chickpea Fattoush

Carbs 16g
Fibre 7.3g
Calories 318 kcal
per serving

This twist on fattoush – the popular Middle Eastern chopped salad – replaces the more usual shards of crisp pitta bread with fibre-filled chickpeas. You can either use the chickpeas straight from the tin or roast them, as here, until crisp to tie in with the salad's signature mix of contrasting textures, flavours and colours. The salad is also good topped with crumbled feta for an added protein element.

Serves 4
Prep: 15 minutes
Cook: 30 minutes

1 tbsp extra virgin olive oil

2 tsp hot smoked paprika

400g/14 oz can chickpeas, drained

6 vine-ripened tomatoes, deseeded and cut into bite-sized chunks

1 small cucumber, quartered lengthways, deseeded and cut into bite-sized chunks

12 radishes, thinly sliced

½ small red onion, diced

2 handfuls roughly chopped mint

2 large handfuls roughly chopped flat-leaf parsley

1 Little Gem (Boston) lettuce, roughly chopped

1 handful almonds, preferably smoked

For the dressing

5 tbsp extra virgin olive oil

2 tsp white wine vinegar

2 tbsp lemon juice, plus finely grated zest ½ unwaxed lemon

1 garlic clove, minced

1 tsp sumac, plus extra to sprinkle

Preheat the oven to 170°C fan/190°C/375°F/gas mark 5.

Line a large baking tray (sheet) with baking (parchment) paper. Mix together the olive oil and paprika in a mixing bowl, then season. Pat the chickpeas dry, removing any loose skins, then add them to the bowl. Turn the chickpeas until coated in the spice oil, then tip them onto the lined baking tray and spread out evenly. Roast for 30 minutes, turning occasionally, or until crisp and golden – they will crisp up further when cooled.

Meanwhile, mix together the dressing ingredients and season with salt and pepper.

Put the tomatoes in a mixing bowl with the cucumber, radishes, onion and three-quarters of the herbs. Spoon over enough of the dressing to coat and toss gently until combined.

Arrange the lettuce on a serving plate and top with the tomato mixture. Scatter over the remaining herbs, chickpeas (save some to snack on as you probably won't want to use all of them) and the almonds, if using. Add a final sprinkling of sumac.

Thai Salmon & Brown Rice Fishcakes

Carbs 22.5g
Fibre 2.4g
Calories 332 kcal
per serving

I'm not one to turn my nose up at canned fish, in fact I prefer it in fishcakes for both its flavour and texture. Perhaps surprisingly, canned salmon is nutritionally on a par with fresh and is a rich source of omega-3 fatty acids and calcium. There are also good carbs and fibre from the brown jasmine rice in this dish, which helps to hold the fishcakes together.

Serves 4
Prep: 20 minutes
Cook: 25 minutes

3 spring onions (scallions), finely chopped

2 lemon grass stalks, outer layers removed, sliced

2 garlic cloves

2.5cm/1 in piece fresh ginger, peeled and thinly sliced

1 tbsp Thai fish sauce

270g/9½ oz/1½ cups cooked and cooled brown jasmine rice (90g/3¼ oz/scant ½ cup dried weight)

2 x 215g/7½ oz cans wild red salmon, drained, skin and large bones removed, flaked

2 red jalapeño chillies, diced

3 kaffir lime leaves, shredded

1 large handful coriander (cilantro), chopped, plus extra to garnish

1 egg white

olive oil, for brushing

200ml/7 fl oz/1 cup coconut milk

juice of 1 large lime

sea salt and black pepper

lime wedges, 100g/3½ oz watercress and ½ cucumber, sliced into ribbons, to serve

Put 2 spring onions in a mini food processor with the lemon grass, 1 garlic clove, the ginger and 2 teaspoons of fish sauce, then blitz to a paste. Scrape the paste into a mixing bowl.

Put two-thirds of the cooked rice in the processor and blend to a coarse paste. Add to the bowl with the lemon grass paste. Add the remaining rice, salmon, half the chilli, the kaffir lime leaves and coriander. Season with salt and pepper and stir in the egg white. Form the mixture into 12 small fishcakes and chill for 20 minutes.

Preheat the oven to 200°C fan/220°C/425°F/gas mark 7.

Line two baking trays (sheets) with baking paper, then lightly oil. Arrange the fishcakes on the trays, brush the tops with oil and cook for 20–25 minutes, turning halfway through cooking, until golden.

Meanwhile, make the coconut dressing. Finely chop the remaining garlic clove and put it in a small saucepan with the coconut milk, lime juice and the remaining chilli, spring onion and fish sauce. Season with pepper and warm gently.

Serve the fishcakes with the coconut dressing, lime wedges, watercress and cucumber alongside and a scattering of extra coriander leaves.

Warm Puy Lentil Salad with Mustard Dressing

Carbs 24.2g
Fibre 7.9g
Calories 374g
per serving

Puy lentils hold their shape better than other types of lentil when cooked, which makes them perfect for more substantial salads, stews or one-pan dishes. They also benefit from a robust dressing like this mustard and garlic one. Serve topped with a poached or fried egg for a deliciously simple meal.

Serves 4
Prep: 10 minutes
Cook: 30 minutes

140g/5 oz/ ¾ cup dried Puy lentils, rinsed

2 tbsp extra virgin olive oil

1 large onion, chopped

4 courgettes (zucchini), quartered lengthways and sliced

3 garlic cloves, finely chopped

2 tbsp finely chopped fresh rosemary

4 good handfuls spinach, tough stalks removed and leaves sliced

4 poached or fried eggs, to serve (optional)

For the dressing

3 tbsp extra virgin olive oil

4 tsp red wine vinegar

1 heaped tsp Dijon mustard

1 small garlic clove, crushed

sea salt and black pepper

Put the lentils in a saucepan and cover generously with water. Bring to the boil, then reduce the heat and simmer for 25–30 minutes until tender. Drain and tip into a shallow serving bowl.

Meanwhile, heat the olive oil in a large sauté pan over a medium-low heat and cook the onion, covered and stirring occasionally, for 10 minutes or until tender. Add the courgettes and cook for a further 5 minutes or until tender and starting to colour. Stir in the garlic, rosemary and spinach and simmer, occasionally turning the spinach with tongs for 2 minutes or until wilted. Add a splash of water to the pan if needed to help the spinach cook evenly.

Mix together all the ingredients for the dressing and add to the pan with the cooked lentils. Season well and stir until combined.

Serve warm or at room temperature topped with a poached or fried egg, if you like.

Crispy Tofu with Relish & Spicy Mayo

Carbs 20.2g
Fibre 2g
Calories 499 kcal
per serving

Rather than going to waste, blitz slightly stale wholewheat bread into breadcrumbs, which will be more nutritious than the processed white ones that you can buy. The tofu is coated in a wholewheat and sesame seed crust, baked in the oven and served with mayo and a crunchy vegetable relish. They are delicious with the Sweet Potato Chips (page 112).

Serves 4
Prep: 25 minutes, plus marinating
Cook: 30 minutes

400g/14 oz firm tofu, drained well
2 tbsp light soy sauce
2 garlic cloves, grated
2.5cm/1 in piece fresh ginger, grated (no need to peel)
40g/1½ oz/scant 1 cup wholewheat breadcrumbs
1 tbsp sesame seeds
2 tbsp cornflour (cornstarch)
1 egg
olive oil, for drizzling
sea salt and black pepper

For the spicy mayonnaise
5 tbsp good-quality mayonnaise
1½ tsp gochujang paste or chilli sauce
juice of 1 lime

To serve
8 radishes, thinly sliced
1 small red onion, thinly sliced
13cm/5 in piece cucumber, quartered lengthways, deseeded and diced
8 Little Gem lettuce leaves

Cut the tofu in half, then cut each piece in half horizontally to make four pieces. Pat dry to remove any excess water. Mix the soy sauce, garlic and ginger in a shallow dish large enough to hold the tofu. Add the tofu, spoon over the marinade, and marinate for 1 hour, occasionally basting the tofu pieces.

Meanwhile, mix together the ingredients for the spicy mayonnaise, using half the lime juice. Mix together the radishes, red onion and cucumber with the remaining lime juice and season with salt. Set aside.

Put the breadcrumbs and sesame seeds in a shallow dish. Put the cornflour in a separate shallow dish and season with salt and pepper. Finally, crack the egg into a shallow bowl and lightly beat with a fork.

Preheat the oven to 180°C fan/200°C/400°F/gas mark 6. Line a baking tray with baking paper and drizzle over some oil.

Dunk the tofu pieces, one at a time, in the cornflour, then the egg and finally the breadcrumb mixture until coated all over. Place on the lined baking tray and repeat until all the tofu is coated in crumbs. Drizzle some oil over the tofu and bake for 25–30 minutes, turning halfway, until golden and crisp.

To serve, place 2 lettuce leaves on top of one another on each serving plate, top with the crispy tofu, a spoonful of spicy mayonnaise and the radish mixture.

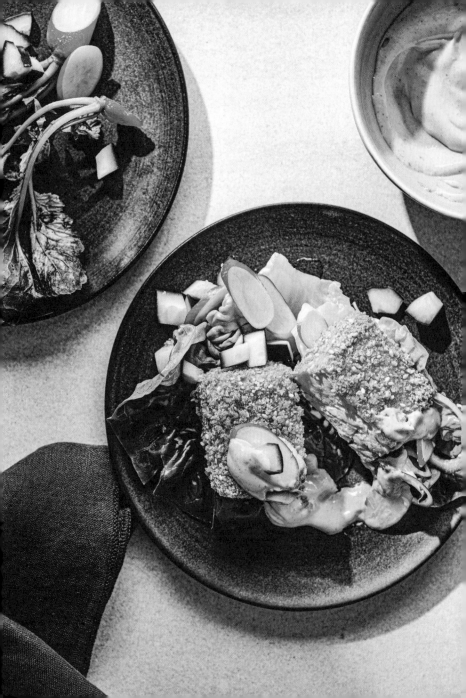

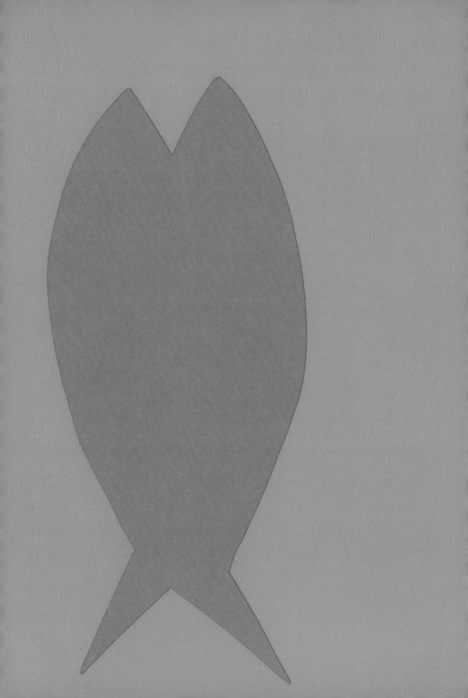

03
Big Plates

Beetroot Spaghetti with Dolcelatte, Walnuts & Chard

Carbs 57.7g
Fibre 11.8g
Calories 641 kcal
per serving

Wholemeal pasta is nutritionally superior to white as it is richer in fibre, iron, zinc, magnesium and selenium, yet visually it's perhaps not so appealing. The addition of beetroot, however, brightens things up, turning the pasta a vibrant pinky-red while also contributing valuable fibre, vitamin C and iron. The chard adds a touch of green, as would beetroot leaves, spinach, kale or cabbage.

Serves 4
Prep: 15 minutes
Cook: 25 minutes

300g/10½ oz wholewheat spaghetti

125g/4½ oz rainbow chard, stalks and leaves separated, then sliced

175g/6 oz cooked beetroots (beets) in natural juice (not vinegar), drained and roughly chopped

75g/2½ oz/⅔ cup walnut pieces

3 tbsp extra virgin olive oil

1 onion, finely chopped

3 garlic cloves, finely chopped

squeeze of lemon juice

125g/4½ oz/½ cup dolcelatte or Gorgonzola cheese, crumbled into small chunks

sea salt and black pepper

Cook the spaghetti in plenty of boiling salted water following the packet instructions.

Meanwhile, steam the chard leaves and stalks, then refresh them under cold running water and set aside.

Purée the beetroot using a stick blender and set aside. Toast the walnuts in a large, dry frying pan (skillet) for 3 minutes, tossing them occasionally until they start to colour. Set aside.

Heat a large sauté pan over a medium heat. Add the oil and onion and sauté for 7 minutes, then add the garlic and cook for a further minute. Add the beetroot purée and cook, stirring, for 2 minutes until reduced slightly.

When the pasta is cooked but still a little al dente, drain, saving 100ml/3½ fl oz/7 tbsp of the cooking water. Add the pasta to the beetroot mixture along with enough of the cooking water to make a light sauce. Turn the pasta to coat it in the sauce, adding more of the cooking water, if needed. Add the chard leaves and stalks, a good squeeze of lemon juice and season with salt and pepper. Warm through briefly.

Spoon the pasta into four large shallow bowls and finish with the toasted walnuts and dolcelatte or Gorgonzola.

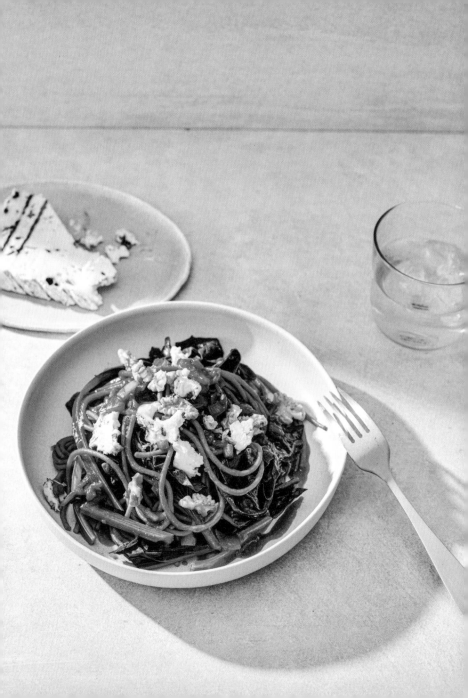

White Bean & Aubergine One-pot with Courgette Tzatziki

Carbs 23.2g
Fibre 10.5g
Calories 274 kcal
per serving

This Mediterranean-style stew is packed with summer vegetables and is given a nutrient boost by the haricot beans, although feel free to add your own favourite bean. You can't beat canned beans for convenience, providing a combination of carbs, fibre and protein, but be mindful of those with added salt as they can be high in sodium. Serve with wholewheat couscous, if liked.

Serves 4
Prep: 20 minutes
Cook: 35 minutes

3 tbsp extra virgin olive oil
1 large onion, roughly chopped
1 large aubergine (eggplant), cut into small chunks
2 courgettes (zucchini), cut into bite-sized chunks
3 garlic cloves, finely chopped
1 tsp fennel seeds
1 red medium-hot chilli, deseeded and finely chopped
2 rounded tbsp tomato purée
4 vine-ripened tomatoes, chopped
400g/14 oz can haricot (cannellini) beans, drained and rinsed
4 long sprigs fresh thyme, leaves picked or 1½ tsp dried
4 long sprigs fresh oregano, leaves picked or 1½ tsp dried
good squeeze of lemon juice

For the courgette tzatziki
150g/5½ oz/scant ¾ cup Greek-style yogurt
1 courgette, coarsely grated
1 garlic clove, grated
1 handful chopped mint
juice of 1 small lemon

Heat a large, heavy-based saucepan over a medium heat. Add the oil, onion and aubergine and cook for 10 minutes, stirring often, until softened – it will look as though there is not enough oil at first, but persist and the aubergine will start to release the oil as it cooks. Stir in the courgettes and garlic and cook for a further 3 minutes, stirring often.

Stir in the fennel seeds, chilli, tomato purée, tomatoes, beans, herbs and 5 tablespoons of water and bring almost to the boil. Reduce the heat to low and simmer, partially covered, for 20 minutes or until the tomatoes have broken down. Add a splash more water if needed. Season with salt and pepper and add a good squeeze of lemon juice.

Meanwhile, mix together all the ingredients for the tzatziki and set aside.

Spoon the stew into four large shallow bowls and serve with the tzatziki on the side.

'Relaxed' Mushroom Lasagne

Carbs 53.4g
Fibre 13.1g
Calories 487 kcal
per serving

This 'relaxed' free-form lasagne is literally tumbled together, rather than assembled in neat even layers. This means it's much quicker and easier to make and uses a smaller quantity of pasta than usual, with the lentils adding extra substance, goodness and fibre. It's perfect with a large green salad.

Serves 4
Prep: 20 minutes
Cook: 45 minutes

200g/7 oz dried wholemeal lasagne sheets

2 tbsp extra virgin olive oil, plus extra for drizzling

1 large onion, finely chopped

1 large celery stick, finely chopped

300g/10½ oz/5½ cups chestnut (cremini) mushrooms, finely chopped

3 large garlic cloves, finely chopped

1 tsp dried thyme

500g/1 lb 2 oz passata (strained tomatoes)

1 tsp dark soy sauce

400g/14 oz can green lentils, drained

125g/4½ oz/½ cup mozzarella cheese, drained, patted dry and torn into chunks

20g/¾ oz/¼ cup Parmesan cheese, finely grated, plus extra to serve

1 handful basil leaves

sea salt and black pepper

Cook the lasagne sheets in boiling salted water in a large, wide saucepan following the packet instructions. Drain and refresh the pasta under cold running water, taking care not to tear the sheets, then immerse them in a shallow dish of cold water to stop them sticking together.

Meanwhile, heat a large, deep, ovenproof sauté pan over a medium heat. Add the oil, onion and celery and cook for 7 minutes, then add the mushrooms, garlic and thyme and cook for 8 minutes or until the mushrooms start to turn golden and any liquid in the pan has evaporated.

Stir in the passata, soy sauce, 100ml/3½ fl oz/7 tbsp water and the lentils and when the sauce starts to bubble, reduce the heat and simmer, partially covered, for 15 minutes until reduced and thickened. Season with salt and pepper to taste.

Preheat the grill to high.

Cut each lasagne sheet in half lengthways then fold them gently into the sauce with a third of the mozzarella. Drizzle extra oil over the top and scatter with the rest of the mozzarella and the Parmesan. Grill for 15 minutes or until the top turns golden. Serve topped with extra Parmesan and the basil leaves.

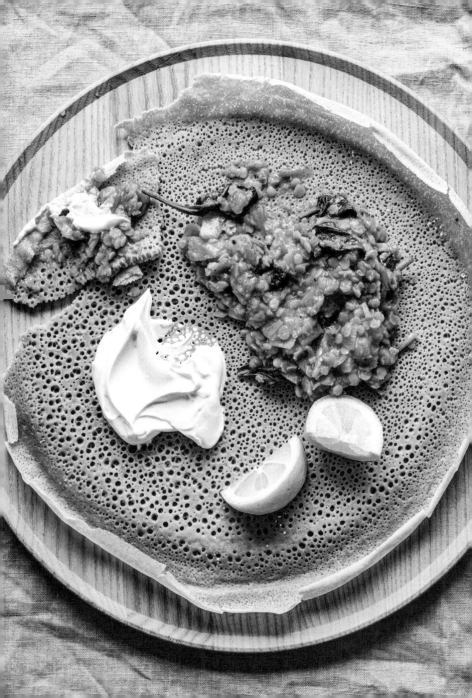

Ethiopian Red Lentil & Tomato Curry

Carbs 40.5g
Fibre 7.5g
Calories 335 kcal
per serving

Based on the traditional Ethiopian lentil dish, *misir wot*, this curry features the wonderfully fragrant spice mix berbere. This aromatic blend of chilli, ginger, garlic, nigella, fenugreek, paprika, cumin, coriander and cardamom imparts an unmistakable depth of flavour as well as benefiting the digestive system. The dish is traditionally served with a fermented flatbread called *injera* made from teff flour, but wholewheat flatbreads or chapattis are good, too.

Serves 4
Prep: 15 minutes
Cook: 35 minutes

20g/¾ oz/scant 2 tbsp butter

1 tbsp extra virgin olive oil

1 large onion, chopped

2 large garlic cloves, finely chopped

5cm/2 in piece ginger, peeled and finely chopped

2 tbsp tomato purée (tomato paste)

6 vine-ripened tomatoes, chopped

1 tbsp berbere spice blend

225g/8 oz/1¼ cups split red lentils, rinsed well

2 bay leaves

800–900ml/28–31 fl oz/3½–scant 4 cups vegetable or chicken stock

100g/3½ oz baby spinach leaves

juice of ½ lemon, plus wedges, to serve

sea salt and black pepper

Greek-style yogurt and wholewheat flatbreads, to serve

Heat a large, heavy-based saucepan over a medium heat. Add the butter, oil and onion and cook for 7 minutes, stirring occasionally, until softened. Add the garlic and ginger and cook for 1 minute, stirring.

Stir in the tomato purée, tomatoes and berbere, then add the lentils, bay leaves and the smaller quantity of stock and bring to the boil. Reduce the heat to low and simmer, partially covered, for 20 minutes until the lentils are tender and the stew has reduced and thickened. Stir in the spinach, season generously with salt and pepper, then stir in the lemon juice. Cook for a further 3 minutes or until the spinach has wilted. Add more stock if necessary.

Serve the stew topped with a good spoonful of yogurt, warmed flatbreads and lemon wedges for squeezing.

Beef & Barley Soup with Winter Greens

Carbs 23.3g
Fibre 5.3g
Calories 342 kcal
per serving

This warming, hearty soup-cum-stew is brimming with goodness. Barley helps to thicken the stock as well as adding valuable minerals and fibre in the form of beta-glucan, which has been found to reduce harmful LDL cholesterol levels in the body and help improve blood sugar control. The small amount of beef is supplemented with plentiful amounts of vegetables.

Serves 4–6
Prep: 20 minutes
Cook: 1½ hours

2 tbsp extra virgin olive oil

400g/14 oz lean beef shin, cut into 1cm/½ in chunks

2 onions, roughly chopped

2 carrots, sliced

2 celery sticks, sliced

3 large garlic cloves, finely chopped

250g/9 oz/5 cups chestnut (cremini) mushrooms, torn into pieces

70g/2½ oz/⅓ cup pearl barley, rinsed well

2 tbsp finely chopped rosemary

2 bay leaves

1.4 litres/48fl oz/6 cups beef stock

150g/5½ oz cavolo nero (Tuscan kale), tough stalks removed, leaves sliced

sea salt and black pepper

Heat a large, heavy-based saucepan over a medium-high heat. Add half the oil and beef and brown all over for 5 minutes. Remove the beef with a slotted spoon and repeat with the remaining beef. Remove from the pan and set aside.

Reduce the heat to medium, pour in the rest of the oil and add the onions, carrots and celery and cook for 5 minutes. Add the garlic and mushrooms and cook for a further 8 minutes until softened.

Return the beef to the pan with the barley, rosemary, bay leaves and stir until combined, then pour in the stock and bring to the boil. Reduce the heat to low and simmer, partially covered with a lid, for 1 hour, stirring occasionally, or until the barley and beef are tender. If the beef is still a bit tough, cook for a further 15 minutes and taste again. Add more stock or water as needed – it should look like a hearty broth, rather than a thick stew.

Stir in the cavolo nero and cook for a further 5 minutes or until wilted and just tender. Remove the bay leaves, season with salt and pepper and serve in large shallow bowls.

Tandoori-style Chicken with Dahl Sauce

Carbs 18.1g
Fibre 2g
Calories 429 kcal
per serving

Spiced red lentils makes a surprisingly good curry sauce when blended until smooth – and it's also an excellent way to encourage non-lentil lovers to give them a try. Fibre-rich lentils pack a powerful punch nutritionally being a good source of both complex carbs and protein. I like to serve this dish with wholemeal chapattis and steamed spinach.

Serves 4
Prep: 20 minutes, plus marinating
Cook: 40 minutes

2½ tbsp tandoori spice mix
2 tsp ground turmeric
3 garlic cloves, crushed
2 tbsp minced fresh ginger
250g/9 oz/1 cup plus 2½ tbsp plain yogurt
juice of 1 lemon
1 tsp sea salt
2 tsp extra virgin olive oil
8 skinless, boneless chicken thighs
sea salt and black pepper
steamed spinach and coriander (cilantro) leaves, to serve

For the dahl sauce
85g/3 oz/scant ½ cup split red lentils, rinsed well
25g/1 oz/2 tbsp butter or ghee
¼–½ tsp dried chilli flakes
2 garlic cloves, crushed
1 tsp garam masala

For the chicken marinade, mix the tandoori spices with half the turmeric, the garlic, ginger, yogurt, half the lemon juice, the salt and oil in a shallow dish. Add the chicken and spoon over the marinade until completely coated. Cover and marinate in the fridge for at least 1 hour, preferably overnight.

Preheat the oven to 200°C fan/220°C/425°F/gas mark 7.

Turn the chicken in the marinade, then spread out in a large roasting tin. Spoon over any leftover marinade and roast for 35–40 minutes, until starting to blacken at the edges.

Meanwhile, make the dahl sauce. Tip the lentils into a pan and cover with 500ml/17 fl oz/2 cups water. Bring to the boil, skimming off any froth that rises to the surface, then reduce the heat to low and simmer, partially covered, for 15 minutes until the lentils are very tender and starting to break down. Using a stick blender, blend the lentil mixture to a smooth sauce.

While the lentils are cooking, melt the butter or ghee in a frying pan (skillet) and add the chilli flakes (starting off with ¼ teaspoon), the garlic and garam masala and cook for 1 minute. Stir the spice butter into the lentils with the remaining turmeric and lemon juice. Season generously with salt and pepper, adding another ¼ teaspoon of chilli flakes, if needed.

Spoon the spinach onto each plate and top with the chicken. Serve with the dahl sauce and a scattering of coriander leaves.

Quick Roast Chicken with White Bean & Rosemary Mash

Carbs 28g
Fibre 10.3g
Calories 601 kcal
per serving

Much as I love potatoes, this herby white bean mash makes a fantastic right-carb alternative. You can either mash the beans roughly with a potato masher so they retain a bit of texture, or blend using a stick blender into a smooth and creamy sauce. Chicken thighs are not only full of flavour, they're much cheaper than breasts – try to buy organic, free-range, if you can.

Serves 4
Prep: 15 minutes
Cook: 35 minutes

6–8 chicken thighs on the bone, skin on

2 red onions, halved and each cut into 6 wedges

1 tbsp extra virgin olive oil

1 large unwaxed lemon, halved

3 bay leaves

2 sprigs fresh rosemary

300g/10½ oz small vine-ripened tomatoes

sea salt and black pepper

For the white bean & rosemary mash

2 x 400g cans cannellini beans, drained and rinsed

270ml/9½ fl oz/scant 1¼ cups whole milk

3 bay leaves

4 garlic cloves, peeled and halved

40g/1½ oz/3 tbsp unsalted butter

2 tsp Dijon mustard

2 tsp finely chopped rosemary

Preheat the oven to 180°C fan/200°C/400°F/gas mark 6.

Season the chicken thighs with salt and pepper and place in a large roasting tin (pan). Toss the onions in the oil and place around the chicken. Squeeze over the lemon juice and cut the halves into chunks and place in the tin. Tuck in the bay leaves and rosemary sprigs. Roast for 20 minutes, then remove the rosemary and add the tomatoes and cook for a further 15 minutes or until the chicken is golden and cooked through.

Meanwhile, make the white bean and rosemary mash. Put all the ingredients, except the rosemary, in a saucepan over a medium heat, stirring occasionally. When it almost starts to bubble, reduce the heat to low and cook, covered with a lid, for 5 minutes. Turn off the heat and set aside for the flavours to infuse while the chicken is roasting. When ready to serve, remove the bay leaf and either mash with a potato masher or blend using a stick blender until smooth and creamy. Season with salt and pepper, stir in the rosemary and warm through.

Serve the chicken with the tomatoes and onions, spooning over any juices from the tin, and the white bean mash on the side.

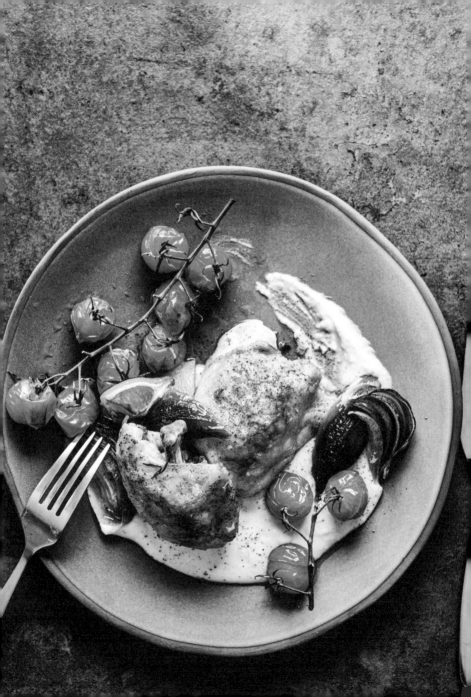

White Fish with Butternut & Ginger Mash

Carbs 21.9g
Fibre 5.9g
Calories 340 kcal
per serving

Mash doesn't have to mean potatoes and it's well worth experimenting with different alternatives – carrot, parsnip, celeriac, Jerusalem artichoke and sweet potato versions are all delicious (or why not try canned beans? See page 88). This golden-hued mash has an Asian feel thanks to the addition of coconut, ginger, chilli and coriander leaves.

Serves 4
Prep: 20 minutes
Cook: 20 minutes

2 tbsp extra virgin olive oil
3cm/1½ in piece fresh ginger, peeled and cut into thin matchsticks
4 thick hake fillets, or other sustainable firm white fish, such as haddock
20g/¾ oz/1½ tbsp butter
sea salt and black pepper
steamed long-stem broccoli and lime wedges, to serve

For the butternut & ginger mash

1kg/1lb 2oz butternut squash, peeled and cut into chunks
4 garlic cloves, peeled and left whole
5cm/2 in piece fresh ginger, peeled and sliced into rounds
2 red jalapeño chillies, deseeded and diced
115ml/3¾ fl oz/scant ½ cup unsweetened drinking coconut milk
juice of ½ lime, plus extra if needed
2 handfuls chopped coriander (cilantro) leaves, plus extra to serve

First make the mash. Put the squash in a saucepan with the garlic and ginger, cover with water and bring to the boil. Reduce the heat and simmer, partially covered, for 10 minutes or until tender. Drain well and pick out the ginger. Return the squash to the hot pan and add half the chilli, most of the coconut milk and the lime juice. Mash until smooth, adding the rest of the coconut milk, if needed. Season with salt and pepper and stir in three-quarters of the coriander leaves. Taste and add more lime juice if needed.

Meanwhile, heat 1 tablespoon of the oil in a large frying pan (skillet) over a medium heat, add the ginger matchsticks and fry for 2 minutes or until crisp and golden. Remove from the pan with a slotted spoon and drain on kitchen paper.

Season the fish with salt and pepper. Add the remaining oil and the butter to the frying pan and heat over a high heat. Place the fish, skin-side down, in the pan, then reduce the heat to medium. Cook for 3–4 minutes until the skin is crisp and golden and you can see the flesh has cooked two-thirds of the way up. Turn the fish over, baste with the buttery oil and cook for a further 2 minutes or until just done and the fish is opaque and flaky.

Warm the mash if need be and spoon onto four serving plates. Top with the broccoli and fish and scatter over the crispy ginger, the remaining chilli and coriander leaves before serving.

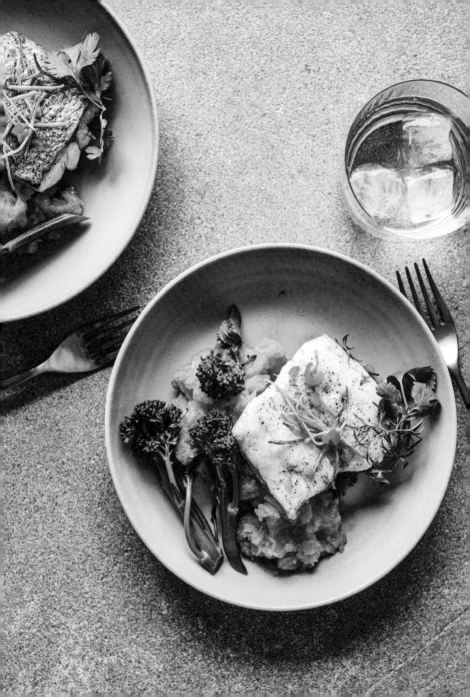

Leek Galette with Sunflower Seed Crust

Carbs 29g
Fibre 8.5g
Calories 596 kcal
per serving

Leeks are joined by spring onions (scallions), spinach and peas in this vegetable-packed, free-form wholewheat tart. It has a nutty spelt crust, with sunflower seeds for a boost of healthy fats, protein, vitamins and minerals. Enjoy with a large tomato and basil salad.

Serves 6

Prep: 20 minutes, plus chilling

Cook: 50 minutes

3 tbsp sunflower seeds

200g/7 oz/1¼ cups wholewheat spelt flour, plus extra for dusting

140g/5 oz/⅔ cup cold unsalted butter, cut into small cubes

2–4 tablespoons chilled water

For the filling

25g/1 oz/2 tbsp unsalted butter

2 leeks, thinly sliced

6 spring onions (scallions), thinly sliced

100g/3½ oz baby leaf spinach

125g/4½ oz/generous 1 cup frozen peas, defrosted

2 eggs, plus 1 extra, beaten, for glazing

3 tbsp double (heavy) cream

100g/3½ oz/scant 1 cup mature Cheddar or Gruyère cheese, grated

sea salt and black pepper

For the pastry, blitz the sunflower seeds in a grinder until finely chopped, then tip into a large mixing bowl with the flour and a large pinch of salt. Using your fingertips, rub in the butter until it forms coarse breadcrumbs. (Alternatively, you can do this in a food processor or mixer.) Stir in the water with a fork, starting with the smaller amount and adding more if needed, then press the mixture together to form a smooth, soft ball of dough. Form the pastry into a disc, then wrap in clingfilm and chill for 30 minutes.

Meanwhile, for the filling, melt the butter in a sauté pan over a medium-low heat, add the leeks and cook for 5 minutes, covered and stirring occasionally, until softened. Add the spring onions and cook for 2 minutes until softened. Stir in the spinach and cook, turning, until wilted, then add the peas to warm through. Tip the vegetables into a bowl and leave to cool. Whisk 2 eggs into the cream in a jug and season with salt and pepper, then stir in the cheese. Pour the mixture into the bowl with the cooled vegetables and stir until combined.

Preheat the oven to 180°C fan/200°C/400°F/gas mark 6. Line a square baking sheet with baking paper. Roll out the pastry on a floured work surface into a 34cm/13½ in circle. Using the rolling pin, carefully lift the pastry onto the baking sheet. Pile the vegetable mixture onto the pastry, leaving a 5cm/2 in border. Carefully fold the edges of the pastry over the outer edge of the filling, pleating it where necessary and leaving the top open. Brush the pastry edge with the beaten egg and bake for 35–40 minutes until cooked.

Mushroom, Kale & Spelt 'Risotto'

Carbs 33.3g
Fibre 8.9g
Calories 447 kcal
per serving

Spelt is an ancient form of wheat and in its wholegrain form has a nutty, chewy, satisfying texture that works well with robust flavours. I've also opted for wholegrain spelt for maximum fibre and nutrient content – think iron, calcium, magnesium and zinc.

Serves 4

Prep: 15 minutes, plus soaking

Cook: 1 hour

20g/¾ oz/²⁄₃ cup dried porcini mushrooms

about 700ml/24 fl oz/3 cups hot good-quality vegetable or chicken stock

3 tbsp extra virgin olive oil

2 onions, roughly chopped

350g/12 oz/6⅓ cups chestnut (cremini) mushrooms, torn into chunks

4 tsp fresh thyme leaves or 2 tsp dried thyme

3 garlic cloves, finely chopped

250g/9 oz/1¼ cups wholegrain spelt, rinsed

2 tsp Dijon mustard

150g/5½ oz pointed green cabbage, finely shredded

150g/5½ oz kale, tough stalks removed, leaves torn into small pieces

40g/1½ oz/⅓ cup walnut halves, toasted and roughly chopped

100g/3½ oz/½ cup crumbly goat's cheese (optional)

sea salt and black pepper

Put the porcini in a small bowl and pour over enough boiled water to just cover them. Leave to soften for 20 minutes, then strain, saving the soaking liquor.

Pour the soaking liquid into the stock to make it up to about 750ml/1¼ pints/3¼ cups. Set aside.

Heat a large, deep sauté pan over a medium heat. Add the oil and onions and cook for 5 minutes, covered, until softened. Add the soaked porcini and chestnut mushrooms and cook for a further 8 minutes or until they start to colour and there is no liquid in the pan. Add the thyme, garlic and spelt and cook, stirring, for 1 minute.

Pour in most of the stock, stir well, then reduce the heat slightly and simmer, partially covered, for 35–40 minutes until the spelt is tender but still retains a chewy texture. Add the mustard, cabbage, kale and extra stock, if needed (you want the consistency to be slightly soupy), then cook for a further 5 minutes or until the leaves are wilted and tender. Season with salt and pepper to taste.

Spoon into four large shallow bowls and top with the walnuts and goat's cheese, if using.

Egg-fried Rice Bowl with Pork

Carbs 48.4g
Fibre 6.3g
Calories 555 kcal
per serving

This take on the Indonesian rice dish, *nasi goreng*, is made with fibre-rich, energy-sustaining brown jasmine rice, pork mince, which you can swap for a vegetarian alternative, and lots of veg. Egg is stirred through towards the end of cooking and the dish is topped with crunchy peanuts, cucumber and radishes just before serving – a complete, comforting meal in a bowl.

Serves 4
Prep: 20 minutes
Cook: 20 minutes

1 tbsp light soy sauce

1½ tbsp tomato purée (tomato paste)

1 tsp shrimp paste (optional)

2 tbsp coconut oil

375g/13 oz free-range pork mince

200g/7 oz pointed cabbage, shredded

1 carrot, coarsely grated

6 spring onions (scallions), green and white parts separated, thinly sliced diagonally

1 red chilli, finely chopped

1 thumb-sized piece fresh ginger, peeled and grated

2 garlic cloves, finely chopped

680g/1 lb 8 oz/generous 5 cups cooked, cooled brown jasmine rice (about 225g/8 oz/generous 1 cup uncooked)

2 large eggs, lightly beaten

juice of ½ lime

9cm/3½ in piece cucumber, quartered, deseeded and diced

8 radishes, thinly sliced

3 tbsp roasted peanuts, roughly chopped

sea salt and black pepper

Mix together the soy sauce, tomato purée and shrimp paste, if using, then set aside.

Heat a wok or large frying pan (skillet) over a high heat. Add half the coconut oil and when hot stir in the pork, breaking it up with the back of a fork. Stir-fry for 10 minutes until the pork starts to turn crisp in places. Transfer to a bowl and set aside.

Add the remaining oil to the wok, then the cabbage, carrot, spring onions (saving half of the green parts), chilli, ginger and garlic and stir-fry for 2–3 minutes until just softened. Return the pork to the wok with the cooked rice and soy mixture. Stir-fry until completely heated through and piping hot.

Push the rice mixture to the edge of the wok, leaving a large well in the middle. Add the eggs and cook, stirring, until scrambled, then fold them into the rice. Add the lime juice and season with salt and pepper to taste. Serve the rice in bowls topped with the cucumber, radishes, reserved spring onions and peanuts.

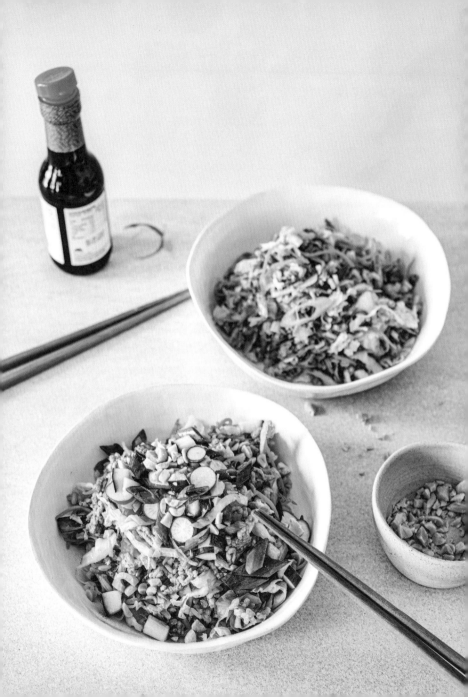

Baked Eggs with Artichokes, Beans & Tomatoes

Carbs 19.4g
Fibre 10.1g
Calories 397 kcal
per serving

This one-pan dish ticks all the right boxes: it provides complex carbs, fibre, healthy fats, protein, a healthy amount of veg, and it tastes great too. To save time, you can make the tomato base in advance and then reheat it briefly before adding the eggs. For a vegan alternative, swap the eggs and goat's cheese for hummus and a handful of toasted almonds or pine nuts spooned on top just before serving.

Serves 4

Prep: 15 minutes

Cook: 30 minutes

3 tbsp extra virgin olive oil

1 large onion, roughly chopped

2 courgettes (zucchini), quartered and cut into small chunks

1 red (bell) pepper, deseeded and thinly sliced

2 large garlic cloves, finely chopped

1½ x 400g/14 oz cans chopped tomatoes

2 tsp dried oregano

2 tsp hot smoked paprika

½ tsp dried chilli flakes

175g/6 oz artichokes from a jar, drained

400g/14 oz can butter beans, drained and rinsed

150g/5½ oz Kalamata olives, stoned

4 eggs

sea salt and black pepper

1 handful chopped flat-leaf parsley leaves and 100g/3½ oz/½ cup goat's cheese, crumbled (optional), to serve

Heat a large, deep sauté pan over a medium heat. Add the oil and onion and cook, covered with a lid, for 5 minutes until softened. Add the courgettes and red pepper and cook for a further 5 minutes, stirring in the garlic in the last minute.

Add the tomatoes, oregano, paprika, chilli, artichokes, beans, olives and 150ml/5 fl oz/scant ²/₃ cup water and when the mixture starts to bubble, reduce the heat slightly and simmer, partially covered, for 15 minutes until reduced and thickened. Season with salt and pepper to taste.

Make four indentations in the sauce, spaced evenly apart, and crack an egg into each one. Cover with a lid and steam-fry the eggs over a medium-low heat for 3–4 minutes until the whites are set but the yolks are still runny. Serve straight away topped with parsley and goat's cheese, if you like.

Mussels with Black Cabbage & Chickpeas

Carbs 37.3g
Fibre 10.3g
Calories 492 kcal
per serving

Mussels have a lot going for them: an impressive nutritional profile, including omega-3 fatty acids and immunity-boosting zinc; they're economical to buy; and are one of our most sustainable seafoods. The chickpeas and wholewheat sourdough provide valuable complex carbs, especially fibre, which help to keep blood sugar levels in check.

Serves 4
Prep: 15 minutes
Cook: 15 minutes

1kg/2 lb 4 oz mussels, cleaned and scrubbed

2 tbsp extra virgin olive oil, plus extra for drizzling

4 shallots, diced

4 garlic cloves, finely chopped, plus 1 whole clove, halved

2 tbsp tomato purée (tomato paste)

½ tsp dried chilli flakes

2 tsp hot smoked paprika

4 tbsp brandy (optional)

400g/14 oz can chickpeas, drained

125g/4½ oz cavolo nero (Tuscan kale), tough stalks removed, leaves torn into bite-sized pieces

juice of ½ lemon

1 handful flat-leaf parsley, roughly chopped

sea salt and black pepper

4 large slices wholewheat sourdough bread, to serve

Check the mussels and discard any with broken shells or that don't close when tapped.

Heat a large, heavy-based saucepan over a medium heat. Add the oil, then the shallots and cook, stirring, for 5 minutes or until tender. Add the garlic and cook for 1 minute. Stir in the tomato purée, chilli, paprika and brandy, if using, and cook for 2 minutes or until reduced and there is no aroma of alcohol. If not using the brandy, add a splash of water.

Meanwhile, toast the bread on a large ridged griddle pan, turning once, until lightly charred in places. Rub one side of each slice of toast with the cut-side of the remaining garlic clove, then drizzle over some olive oil.

Pour 400ml/14 fl oz/1¾ cups water into the pan and add the chickpeas and cavolo nero and cook for 2 minutes or until the cabbage has wilted. Tip in the mussels, increase the heat to medium-high and cook, covered with the lid, shaking the pan occasionally, for 4–5 minutes or until the mussels have opened and have heated through.

Using a large slotted spoon, scoop out the mussels into four large shallow bowls. Taste the cooking liquor, add the lemon juice and season with salt and pepper, then ladle it over the mussels and top with the parsley. Serve with the garlic toasts.

Spiced Roasted Winter Vegetables with Lime Raita

Carbs 45.5g
Fibre 17.6g
Calories 509 kcal
per serving

Loaded with fresh veg, this fibre-rich, nutrient-dense one-pan meal doesn't need any extras. That said, if you wish to up the protein content, you could add cubes of smoked tofu, paneer or halloumi to the mix at the same time as the cauliflower.

Serves 4
Prep: 20 minutes
Cook: 40 minutes

1 small butternut squash, weighing about 650g/1 lb 7 oz, peeled, deseeded and cut into 2.5cm/1 in chunks

3 parsnips, cut into batons

2 red onions, each cut into 6 wedges

400g/14 oz can chickpeas, drained

5 tbsp extra virgin olive oil

2 tsp ground turmeric

1 tbsp cumin seeds

1 tbsp coriander seeds, crushed

1 tbsp garam masala

300g/10½ oz cauliflower, broken into small florets

250g/9 oz Brussels sprouts, peeled

sea salt and black pepper

1 handful toasted flaked almonds and coriander (cilantro) leaves, to serve

For the lime raita

250g/9 oz/1 cup plus 2½ tbsp plain yogurt

2 garlic cloves, crushed

finely grated zest of 1 and juice of 2 unwaxed limes

Preheat the oven to 180°C fan/200°C/400°F/gas mark 6.

Put the squash, parsnips, onions and chickpeas in a large bowl. Pour over 3 tablespoons of the oil and turn the veg with your hands until coated. Tip into a large roasting tin (pan), or use 2 smaller ones, and roast for 20 minutes, turning once.

Meanwhile, mix the remaining oil with the spices and season well with salt and pepper.

After 20 minutes, add the cauliflower and sprouts to the tin(s). Spoon over the spiced oil, add a splash of water and turn until everything is combined. Return the tin(s) to the oven for a further 20 minutes or until the vegetables are tender and starting to colour and caramelize in places.

Meanwhile, make the lime raita. Mix together the yogurt, garlic and lime juice and season with salt and pepper.

Before serving, top the roasted vegetables with the lime zest, almonds and coriander leaves and serve with the raita on the side.

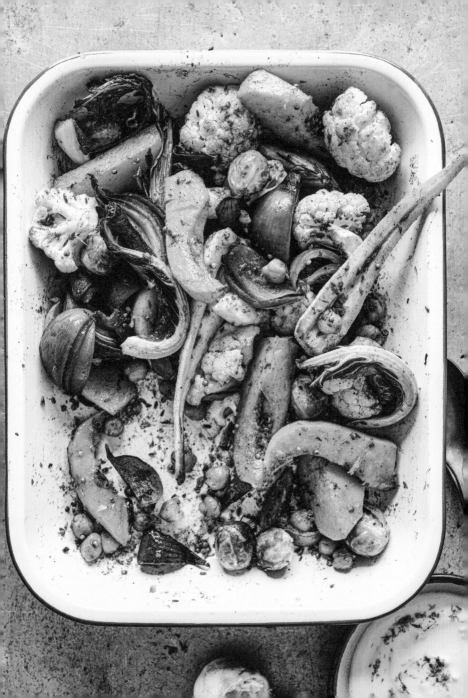

04

On the Side

Orange & Pistachio Quinoa Salad

Carbs 20.1g
Fibre 4.6g
Calories 234 kcal
per serving

Fresh and fragrant, this refreshing salad is a combination of herbs, vegetables, sprouted broccoli and quinoa with a lively citrus dressing. Carb-, protein- and fibre-rich quinoa is also a good source of vital minerals, including iron, magnesium, potassium and zinc.

Serves 4
Prep: 15 minutes
Cook: 15 minutes

125g/4½ oz/¾ cup multi-coloured quinoa, rinsed

1 shallot, diced

1 handful chopped mint

2 handfuls chopped flat-leaf parsley

1 fennel bulb, diced and fronds reserved

1 large handful broccoli sprouts

40g/1½ oz/⅓ cup unsalted shelled pistachios

For the orange dressing
juice of 1 orange
2 tbsp extra virgin olive oil
2 tbsp sherry vinegar
sea salt and black pepper

Put the quinoa in a small saucepan and cover with 400ml/14 fl oz/1¾ cups water. Bring to the boil, then reduce the heat slightly and simmer, partially covered with a lid, for 15 minutes or until tender. Drain if necessary, then leave the quinoa in a serving bowl to cool.

Meanwhile, mix together all the ingredients for the dressing and season with salt and pepper to taste.

When the quinoa is cool, add the shallot, herbs and fennel and toss gently until combined. Pour over enough of the dressing to lightly coat and toss again. Serve topped with the broccoli sprouts, fennel fronds and pistachios. Let everyone help themselves to any remaining dressing.

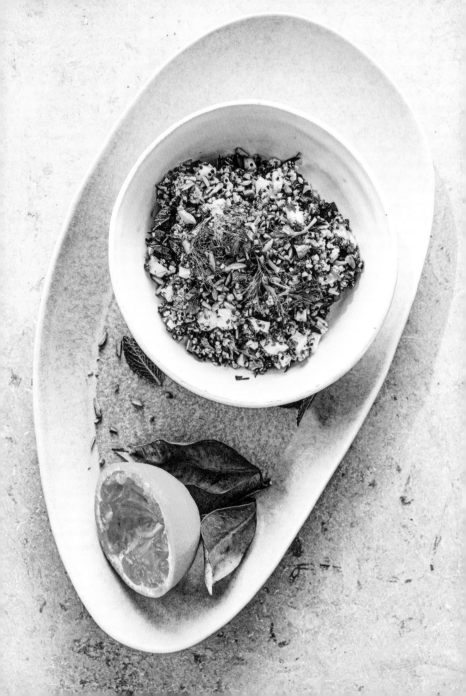

Mixed Cabbage Slaw with Toasted Seeds

Carbs 18.9g
Fibre 7.6g
Calories 298 kcal
per serving

A celebration of brassicas, this is the perfect vegetable side to grilled or roast chicken, fish or meat-free alternatives. I prefer a slaw with a dressing that gently coats the vegetables, rather than drowning them as with some shop-bought options, so the flavour of the veg sings through. This slaw comes with the added nutritional bonus of green lentils and seeds.

Serves 4

Prep: 15 minutes

125g/4½ oz red cabbage, shredded

125g/4½ oz white cabbage, shredded

75g/2½ oz Brussels sprouts, outer leaves removed and shredded

2 carrots, coarsely grated

6 tbsp cooked green lentils

2 tbsp sunflower seeds, toasted

For the dressing

125g/4½ oz/scant ⅔ cup plain yogurt

juice of ½ lemon

1 heaped tsp wholegrain mustard

2 tbsp good-quality mayonnaise

sea salt and black pepper

Mix together all the ingredients for the dressing and season with salt and pepper.

Put the red and white cabbage, sprouts, carrots and lentils in a serving bowl. Spoon over the dressing and turn the vegetables gently until coated. Top with the sunflower seeds just before serving.

Courgette Fries

Carbs 11.8g
Fibre 1.3g
Calories 207 kcal
per serving

With their crunchy cheesy coating, these vegetable fries make a welcome alternative to the usual potato version, and are oven-baked for convenience and health. It's worth trying other vegetables, too. I've given the option of cauliflower and carrot, but you could also use parsnip and celeriac.

Serves 4

Prep: 10 minutes

Cook: 30 minutes

4 tbsp instant polenta (cornmeal)

55g/2 oz/½ cup Parmesan cheese, finely grated

3 courgettes (zucchini), halved crossways, then cut lengthways into batons

2 eggs, lightly beaten

extra virgin olive oil, for drizzling

sea salt and black pepper

Preheat the oven to 180°C fan/200°C/400°F/gas mark 6. Line a baking tray (sheet) with baking (parchment) paper.

Mix together the polenta and Parmesan in a shallow bowl, then season with salt and pepper.

Pat the courgettes dry with kitchen paper. Dunk them, one by one, in the beaten egg using one hand, then the polenta mixture using the other hand until completely coated. Using separate hands for the coating process means you don't get all sticky and messy. Place the coated courgettes on the lined baking tray.

Drizzle olive oil over the courgettes and roast for 25–30 minutes, turning once, until golden and crisp.

Variations

Cut 1 small cauliflower into florets, then dunk into the egg and then the polenta mixture. Drizzle with oil and roast following the instructions above.

Cut 3 carrots into batons, then dunk into the egg and then the polenta mixture. Drizzle with oil and roast following the instructions above.

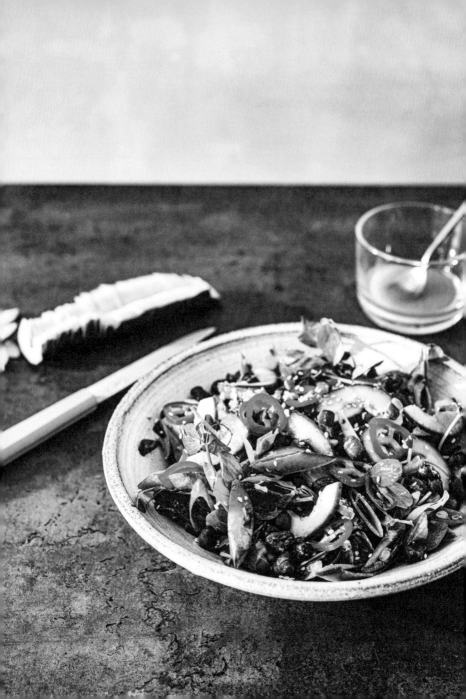

Aduki Bean Salad
with Ginger Sesame Dressing

Carbs 15g
Fibre 6.2g
Calories 176 kcal
per serving

A staple of macrobiotic diets, aduki beans are believed to support the kidneys, reproductive system and bladder. They are also a good source of B vitamins, magnesium, manganese, iron and potassium and are said to be easier to digest than other types of bean, which is a real bonus if you find pulses harsh on the digestive system.

Serves 4

Prep: 15 minutes

400g/14 oz can aduki (adzuki) beans, drained and rinsed

13cm/5 in piece cucumber, quartered lengthways, deseeded and diced

3 spring onions (scallions), thinly sliced diagonally

60g/2 oz sugar snap peas, sliced diagonally

100g/3½ oz pea shoots

1 medium-hot red chilli, deseeded and thinly sliced

2 tsp toasted sesame seeds

For the ginger & sesame dressing

2 tbsp toasted sesame oil

juice of 1 large lime

1.5cm/⁵/₈ in piece fresh ginger, peeled and finely grated

sea salt and black pepper

Mix together all the ingredients for the dressing and season with salt and pepper to taste.

Put all the ingredients for the salad, except the chilli and sesame seeds, into a serving bowl. Pour over the dressing just before serving and toss gently until combined. Scatter over the chilli and sesame seeds.

Roasted Chestnut Salad with Garlic Dressing

Carbs 25.2g
Fibre 10.5g
Calories 236 kcal
per serving

This wintery version of the classic Tuscan panzanella salad uses chestnuts instead of the more usual bread croûtons. Fibre-rich chestnuts are a valuable source of B vitamins, which help the body convert food into energy, along with iron, zinc and calcium for strong bones and teeth.

Serves 4

Prep: 20 minutes

Cook: 40 minutes

350g/12 oz celeriac (celery root), peeled and cubed

2 red onions, halved and each cut into 6 wedges

4 garlic cloves, left whole

400g/14 oz small vine-ripened tomatoes

150g/5½ oz cooked chestnuts, halved

100g/3½ oz kale, tough stalks removed, leaves torn into bite-sized pieces

2 handfuls flat-leaf parsley

For the dressing

3 tbsp extra virgin olive oil, plus extra for roasting

2 tsp Dijon mustard

4 tsp raw apple cider vinegar

sea salt and black pepper

Preheat the oven to 180°C fan/200°C/400°F/gas mark 6.

Put the celeriac, onions and garlic in a large roasting tin (pan), drizzle over some oil and mix with your hands until combined. Roast for 20 minutes, then remove the garlic cloves if soft when pressed and set aside.

Add the tomatoes and chestnuts to the tin and season with salt and pepper. Mix all the ingredients until combined, then cook for a further 20 minutes until the vegetables are tender and golden in places.

Meanwhile, make the dressing. Squeeze the roasted garlic out of its papery skin into a small bowl, add the olive oil and mash using the back of a fork. Mix in the mustard and vinegar and season with salt and pepper.

Put the kale on a large serving dish, drizzle over a little oil and rub the leaves with your fingers until softened slightly. Add half the parsley and the roasted vegetables and spoon over the dressing, then toss gently until combined. Scatter over the remaining parsley before serving.

Bulgur & Quinoa Spiced Tomato Pilaf

Carbs 39.1g
Fibre 6.7g
Calories 348 kcal
per serving

Unlike most plant-based proteins, quinoa is a complete protein, which means it contains all of the nine essential amino acids that the body cannot produce on its own. Both quinoa and bulgur wheat are rich in fibre, folate, calcium, magnesium, thiamine and niacin. They come together beautifully in this simple pilaf, which makes a nutritious side, but can be turned into a more substantial meal with the addition of seafood, chicken, poached or fried eggs, tofu or a crumbly goat's or sheep's cheese.

Serves 4
Prep: 10 minutes
Cook: 30 minutes

2 tbsp extra virgin olive oil
1 large onion, roughly chopped
2 garlic cloves, finely chopped
1 tbsp harissa paste
2 tbsp tomato purée (tomato paste)
1 tsp ground turmeric
200g/7 oz/generous 1 cup bulgur wheat and quinoa mix, rinsed
550ml/19 fl oz/scant 2½ cups hot vegetable stock
150g/5½ oz baby spinach leaves
good squeeze of lemon juice
sea salt and black pepper
40g/1½ oz/⅓ cup unsalted shelled pistachios, roughly chopped (optional), to serve

Heat a large, deep sauté pan over a medium heat. Add the oil and onion and cook, stirring regularly, for 8 minutes until softened. Add the garlic and cook for a further minute.

Stir in the harissa, tomato purée, turmeric and bulgur/quinoa mix, then pour over the stock. Bring to a gentle bubble, then reduce the heat to low, and simmer, covered with a lid, for 15 minutes or until the grains are almost cooked.

Just before the grains are ready and there is still a little liquid in the pan, fold in the spinach, replace the lid and cook for a further 3 minutes or until wilted. Add a good squeeze of lemon juice, season with salt and pepper and stir until combined. Serve scattered with pistachios, if using.

New Potato, Radish & Watercress Salad with Feta

Carbs 21.1g
Fibre 3.6g
Calories 199 kcal
per serving

Potatoes definitely don't have to be a no-no when choosing right carbs. Interestingly, cooked and cooled potatoes are high in resistant starch (see page 18), which has been found to pass through the body in much the same way as fibre and so doesn't cause a spike in blood sugar levels. And the potatoes come with their nutritious skins on, too.

Serves 4
Prep: 15 minutes
Cook: 15 minutes

500g/1 lb 2 oz new potatoes in their skins, scrubbed

100g/3½ oz radishes, thinly sliced into rounds

½ cucumber, quartered, deseeded and diced

5 spring onions (scallions), thinly sliced

100g/3½ oz watercress, torn into small sprigs

1 tbsp extra virgin olive oil or hemp oil

juice of ½ lemon

1 large handful mint leaves

1 handful dill sprigs

100g/3½ oz/scant ½ cup feta cheese, crumbled

sea salt and black pepper

Cook the potatoes in plenty of boiling salted water for 12–15 minutes or until tender. Drain and leave to cool to room temperature.

Just before serving, put the potatoes in a serving bowl with the radishes, cucumber, spring onions and watercress.

Mix together the olive oil and lemon juice and season with salt and pepper. Pour the dressing into the bowl and mix gently until everything is combined. Scatter over the herbs and feta and serve.

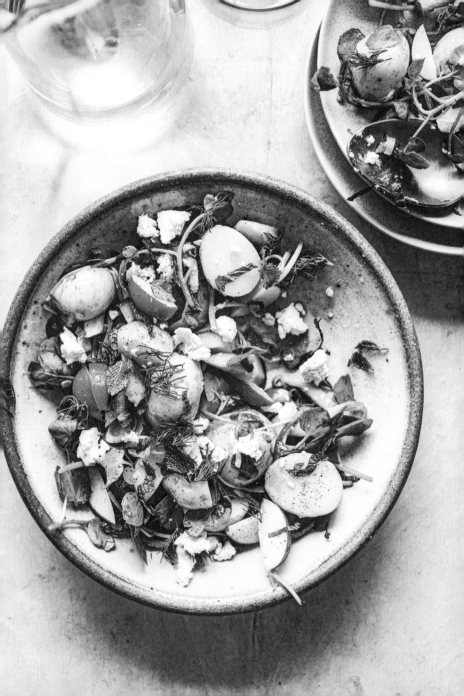

Sweet Potato Chips with Peanuts & Garlic Mayo

Carbs 14.1g
Fibre 2.2g
Calories 361 kcal
per serving

Who doesn't love chips? These pimped-up roast sweet potato chips have slightly more fibre and have a lower GI (see page 12) than regular white potatoes. They are also rich in the antioxidant beta-carotene, the absorption of which is enhanced by the oil. What's more, the protein-packed nuts have been found to help slow the absorption and digestion of the carbs in the sweet potato. Win-win.

Serves 4
Prep: 10 minutes
Cook: 35 minutes

55g/2 oz/½ cup unsalted peanuts
4 small sweet potatoes, skin on and cut into long, thin wedges
1–2 tbsp extra virgin olive oil
1 handful coriander (cilantro) leaves
1 handful mint leaves
1 red jalapeño chilli, thinly sliced
sea salt and black pepper

For the garlic mayo
1 head of garlic
oil, for drizzling
100g/3½ oz/ generous ⅔ cup good-quality mayonnaise
good squeeze of lemon juice

Preheat the oven to 180°C fan/200°C/400°F/gas mark 6. While the oven is heating up, roast the peanuts on a baking tray (sheet) in the bottom of the oven for 10 minutes, turning occasionally, until starting to colour. Leave to cool, then roughly chop.

Put the sweet potato chips in a large bowl with 1 tablespoon of the oil and season with salt and pepper. Turn them with your hands until coated in the oil, adding the rest of the oil if needed. Roast for 30–35 minutes, turning halfway through cooking, until cooked.

Meanwhile, make the garlic mayo. Cut a sliver off the top of the garlic head, drizzle a little oil over, wrap in foil and roast at the same time as the potatoes for 20–30 minutes until the cloves are soft when pressed. Squeeze the garlic out of their papery casings, add a good squeeze of lemon juice and mash with the back of a fork. Stir in the mayonnaise and season to taste.

Serve the sweet potatoes topped with the roasted peanuts, herbs and chilli with the garlic mayo on the side.

Simple Chickpea Mash

Carbs 19.6g
Fibre 7.3g
Calories 212 kcal
per serving

Beans make a great high-fibre, protein- and complex-carb-rich mash – nutritionally a great all-rounder. Chickpeas are used here, but cannellini and butter (lima) beans are also good. For a richer-tasting mash, use milk – dairy or non-dairy – instead of water.

Serves 4
Prep: 10 minutes
Cook: 10 minutes

2 tbsp extra virgin olive oil, plus extra for drizzling
3 shallots, diced
2 garlic cloves, finely chopped
2 x 400g/14 oz cans chickpeas, drained
1 handful chopped flat-leaf parsley
sea salt and black pepper

Put a saucepan over a medium heat. Add the oil and shallots and cook, stirring, for 5 minutes or until softened. Reduce the heat slightly, add the garlic and cook for a minute.

Add the chickpeas and 100ml/3½ fl oz/7 tbsp water to the pan and cook, stirring occasionally, for 5 minutes or until warmed through. Mash with a potato masher, adding more water if needed to make a coarse purée. Season with salt and pepper to taste, and warm through if needed. Serve topped with an extra drizzle of olive oil and the parsley.

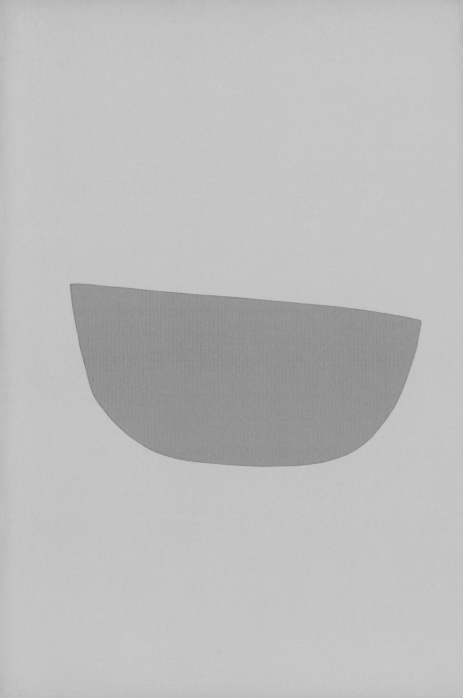

05
Sweet
Treats &
Bakes

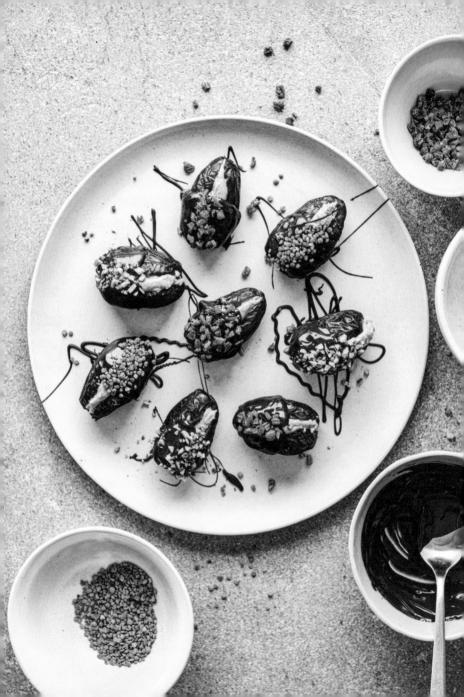

Chocolate & Almond Butter-stuffed Dates

Carbs 21.5g
Fibre 3.2g
Calories 241 kcal
per serving

Reminiscent of a well-known chocolate bar, this healthier version comes with no added sugar. Dates may be sweet – not forgetting delicious – but they are also a good source of nutrients, such as fibre, calcium, magnesium, copper, iron and vitamin B6.

Makes 12
Prep: 15 minutes
Cook: 25 minutes

100g/3½ oz/generous ½ cup dark chocolate (at least 70% cocoa solids), broken into even-sized pieces

12 Medjool dates

chopped unsalted pistachios, dried bee pollen and freeze-dried berries, to decorate (optional)

For the almond nut butter

125g/4½ oz/generous 1 cup almonds

100g/3½ oz/scant 1 cup hazelnuts

1 tbsp extra virgin coconut oil

pinch of sea salt

Start by making the almond nut butter. Preheat the oven to 150°C fan/170°C/325°F/gas mark 3. Line a large baking tray (sheet) with baking (parchment) paper. Spread the almonds and hazelnuts out on the baking tray and bake for 15–20 minutes, turning halfway through cooking, until they start to colour and smell toasted. Leave to cool, then set aside 25g/1 oz/¼ cup of the almonds. Tip the rest of the nuts into a mini food processor or blender. Add the coconut oil and salt and blend until almost smooth and creamy. You may need to scrape the mixture down, once or twice so everything blends evenly. Scoop the nut butter into a jar – you will have more than you need to stuff the dates. Roughly chop the reserved almonds and set aside.

Melt the chocolate in a heatproof bowl placed over a bowl of gently simmering water – don't let the bottom of the bowl touch the water. When the chocolate has melted, carefully remove the bowl from the pan and let it sit for a minute or two to cool slightly.

Make a slit along the length of each date, open out each one and remove the central stone. Place a teaspoonful of the nut butter in the middle and press the two halves of the date together. Repeat with all the dates.

Next, carefully dunk each date into the melted chocolate until coated all over and place on a lined baking tray. Scatter the reserved chopped almonds on top (or decorate with pistachios, bee pollen and freeze-dried berries, if preferred) and leave in a cool place for the chocolate to set. Store in an airtight container in a cool place for up to a week, if they last that long!

Banana & Peanut Butter Ice Cream

Carbs 22.4g
Fibre 2.7g
Calories 427 kcal
per serving

While bananas may be a no-no for some on a low-carb diet, I like to think that they can play a healthy part of good-carb eating. Their natural sweetness means that this simple ice cream needs no added refined sugar, plus it has been suggested that freezing the bananas increases levels of resistant starch (see page 18), which is a form of fibre that helps to feed good bacteria in the gut. The protein in the peanuts also slows down the absorption of the carbs in the bananas, producing a smaller rise in blood sugar.

Serves 4
Prep: 10 minutes, plus freezing

4 just-ripe bananas, peeled
2 tbsp crunchy or smooth peanut butter
6 tbsp thick double (heavy) cream
1 tsp ground cinnamon
pinch of sea salt
3 tbsp roasted unsalted peanuts, roughly chopped

Break each banana into three pieces, place in a resealable freezer bag and freeze until firm.

Remove the bananas from the freezer and leave to soften very slightly – this will make them easier to blend. Put them in a food processor or heavy-duty blender and process until almost smooth. Add the peanut butter, cream, cinnamon and salt, then blend briefly until combined.

Spoon the ice cream into four small glasses or bowls and top with the peanuts. Serve straightaway.

Spiced Melon with Coconut

Carbs 4.5g
Fibre 1.5g
Calories 104 kcal
per serving

Based on the Indian dessert, *rasayana*, this couldn't be simpler to make and features one of the best low-carb fruits, melon. Traditionally, the coconut is sweetened with palm sugar, but the spices and lime lend enough flavour to eliminate the need for any extra sweetness.

Serves 4

Prep: 10 minutes

1 small cantaloupe melon, chilled, cut into wedges and deseeded

½ tsp ground ginger, plus extra to finish

½ tsp freshly ground nutmeg, plus extra to finish

finely grated zest and juice of 1 large unwaxed lime

200ml/7 fl oz/scant 1 cup coconut milk

mint leaves, to decorate

Slice the melon away from the skin and cut the flesh into bite-sized chunks. Chill the melon if not serving it straightaway.

Stir the spices and lime juice into the coconut milk and divide it between four shallow bowls. Add the melon and finish with an extra sprinkling of ginger, nutmeg, lime zest and a few mint leaves.

Grilled Nectarines with Tahini Cream

Carbs 12.3g
Fibre 3.1g
Calories 252 kcal
per serving

Simplicity itself, this is my kind of pudding. There's no need for any added sugar, the ripe nectarines are all you require. The sauce is made with tahini, a wonderfully versatile ingredient that lends itself to both savoury and sweet dishes. Made from toasted, ground hulled sesame seeds, this star addition is a good source of omega-3 fatty acids, protein, iron, calcium and vitamins B and E.

Serves 4
Prep: 10 minutes
Cook: 10 minutes

50g/1½ oz/scant ½ cup pecans
4 ripe nectarines (but not too soft), halved and stoned
mild-tasting olive oil, for brushing

For the tahini cream
250g/9 oz/1 cup plus 2½ tbsp Greek-style yogurt or dairy-free alternative
1 heaped tbsp tahini
1 tsp vanilla extract
½ tsp ground cinnamon, plus extra for sprinkling
splash of milk of your choice (optional)

To make the tahini cream, mix together all the ingredients in a bowl until combined. Taste and add more tahini, if needed. Add a splash of milk if the cream looks too thick.

Toast the pecans in a large, dry frying pan (skillet) over a medium-low heat for 5 minutes, turning once, until they start to colour. Leave to cool then roughly chop.

Pat the cut sides of each nectarine with kitchen paper and brush lightly with oil. Heat a griddle pan over a high heat and place the nectarines cut-side down in the pan. Cook for 2–3 minutes, turning them 90 degrees halfway through cooking to get a criss-cross pattern, if liked. Flip the nectarines over and cook for a further 2 minutes or until softened but not collapsing.

Serve the nectarines warm with a good spoonful of the tahini cream on the side and a scattering of pecans and cinnamon.

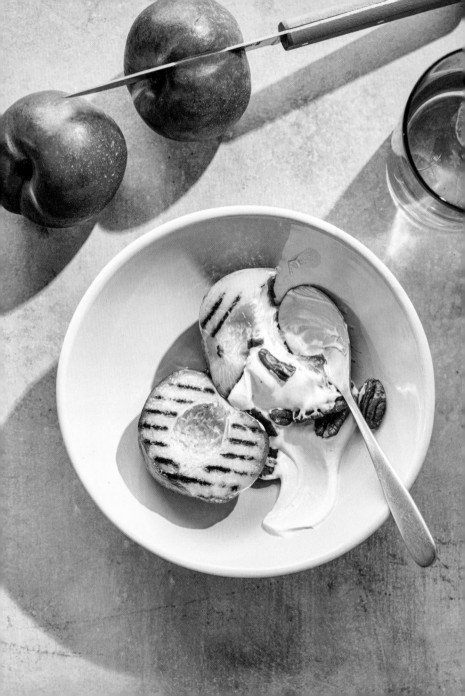

Sweet Potato Fritters
with Strawberries

Carbs 21.9g
Fibre 4.8g
Calories 263 kcal
per serving

Sweet potatoes – in their high-fibre skins – make seriously good fritters. It may come as a surprise to find the root vegetable as part of a dessert, but their natural sweetness combined with the mixed spice and the strawberries means there's no need for any added refined sugar. You could also try carrot or parsnip fritters.

Serves 4
Prep: 15 minutes, plus standing
Cook: 20 minutes

300g/10 oz sweet potatoes,
coarsely grated

2 eggs

2 tsp mixed spice

1 tsp vanilla extract

pinch of sea salt

unsalted butter or extra virgin
coconut oil, for frying

To serve

250g/9 oz strawberries, hulled,
halved or quartered if large

toasted nuts of your choice

coconut or Greek-style yogurt

Squeeze the sweet potatoes in a clean tea towel to remove any excess moisture.

Crack the eggs into a mixing bowl and whisk with the mixed spice, vanilla and salt until combined, then stir in the sweet potatoes.

Heat a large frying pan over a high heat. Reduce the heat to medium and add enough butter or coconut oil to lightly coat the base. Place heaped tablespoons of the sweet potato mixture into the pan and gently flatten with a spatula to make a thin fritter, about 7cm/2¾ in diameter. Cook 4 fritters at a time for 2 minutes on each side or until crisp and golden. Drain on kitchen paper and keep warm in a low oven while you make the remaining fritters, about 16 in total.

Serve the fritters with the strawberries, a scattering of nuts and a good spoonful of yogurt on the side.

Rye & Oatcakes

Carbs 9.6g
Fibre 1.6g
Calories 94 kcal
per oatcake

Many of us don't get enough fibre in our diets (see page 16) and these mixed-grain coarse oatcakes are an easy way to increase intake of both the soluble and insoluble fibre. Eat them plain or serve topped with cheese, pâté or hummus.

Makes 20

Prep: 20 minutes

Cook: 25 minutes

150g/5½ oz/about 1 cup medium oatmeal

50g/1¾ oz/scant ⅓ cup rye flour, plus extra for dusting

100g/3½ oz/generous 1 cup jumbo oats

1 tsp sea salt

½ tsp bicarbonate of soda

2 tbsp sunflower seeds

75g/2½ oz/6 tbsp unsalted butter, melted

Preheat the oven to 160°C fan/180°C/350°F/gas mark 4. Line a large baking sheet with baking (parchment) paper.

Put all the dry ingredients into a large mixing bowl and stir until combined. Pour in the melted butter and stir with a fork until everything is combined. Add 100ml/3½ fl oz/ 7 tbsp water, stir well, then form the mixture into a soft, slightly sticky ball of dough.

Turn the dough out onto a lightly floured work surface and flatten the top slightly. Roll out the dough until about 3mm/⅛ in thick. Using a 6cm/2½ in round cookie cutter, stamp out 20 oatcakes, re-rolling any trimmings as necessary.

Arrange slightly spaced out on the baking sheet and prick the tops with a fork. Bake for 20 minutes, then turn over and cook for a further 5 minutes until crisp and slightly golden. Transfer to a wire rack to cool. They will keep for up to 5 days in an airtight container.

'Sleepless' Spelt Bread

Carbs 40.7g
Fibre 8.5g
Calories 228 kcal
per 100g

Spelt is an ancient type of wheat with a lovely nutty flavour and is generally more tolerated by those who have difficulty eating wheat flour. This slow-rise bread – you could call it a cheat's sourdough – uses an overnight starter, hence the name, which not only enhances the flavour of the bread, but also makes it is easier to digest, so there is less likelihood of bloating. Slow fermentation has also been found to enable nutrients in the bread, such as magnesium, zinc, iron and B vitamins, to be more readily absorbed in the body.

Makes 2 loaves

Prep: 25 minutes, plus overnight rising and 2 hours proving

Cook: 40 minutes

1kg/2 lb 4 oz/6 cups strong wholewheat spelt bread flour, plus extra for dusting

5g/⅛ oz dried yeast

1 tbsp sea salt

extra virgin olive oil, for greasing

The day before you bake the bread, mix the flour, yeast and salt together in a large mixing bowl and make a well in the centre. Gradually, pour in 650–700ml/22–24 fl oz/generous 2½–3 cups lukewarm water, starting off with the smaller quantity and adding more if needed. Stir with a fork and then with your fingers to make a soft ball of dough.

Tip the dough out on to a lightly floured work surface and knead for 10–15 minutes until it is smooth and elastic – it should spring back when pressed with a finger. Shape the dough into a ball and place in a lightly oiled clean mixing bowl. Cover with clingfilm (plastic wrap) and leave to rise overnight (about 10 hours) at room temperature – it can be left for up to 18 hours – until doubled in size.

The next day, line and flour 2 baking trays (sheets). Cut the dough in half in the bowl and carefully tip the dough out onto the trays, taking care not to lose too much air. (Alternatively, place the dough in 2 x 900g/2 lb loaf tins.) Shape each ball of dough into a round. Cover with clean tea towels and leave to prove for about 2 hours or until doubled in size.

Preheat the oven to 200°C fan/220°C/425°F/gas mark 7. Dust the loaves with flour and slash with a utility knife. Pour some cold water into a roasting tin and place in the bottom of the oven – this will create steam and gives the bread a good crust. Bake for 35–40 minutes until golden and the loaves sound hollow when tapped on the bottom. Leave the bread to cool completely on a wire rack. The bread will keep for up to 5 days – you could freeze one of the loaves for later use.

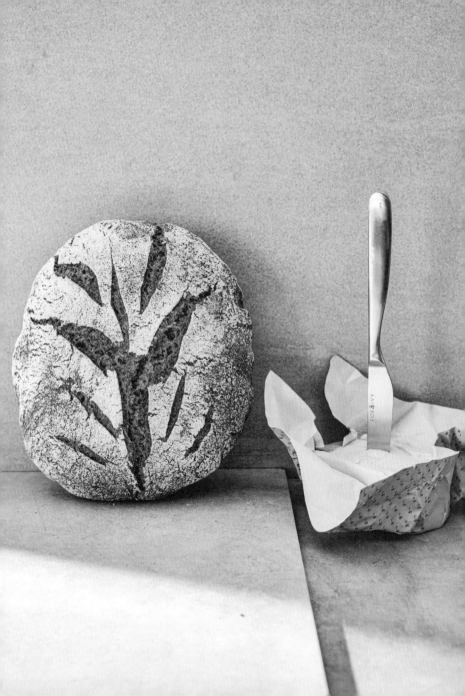

Index

Acknowledgements

A great part of this book was created through lockdown, so it feels a real achievement to finish it, let alone for it to reach the bookshelves, and I have to thank a great team of people for their contribution to getting it over the final hurdle. Firstly, my heartfelt thanks to Stephanie Milner and Katie Cowan for their enthusiasm and interest in my idea in the early stages. My gratitude extends to the team at Pavilion – Helen Lewis, for taking up the mantle, designer, Laura Russell, and to Sophie Allen, project editor – it has been such a pleasure to work with you and thank you. Thanks also to editor, Vicky Orchard, and proofreader, Stephanie Evans. The photographers Liz and Max at Haarala Hamilton, you've been stars as usual – thank you so much. And Valerie Berry, well what can I say – fab styling! Last but not least, I have to thank Rachel Vere for prop styling – it couldn't have been an easy job to do during this period of time. Thank you all!